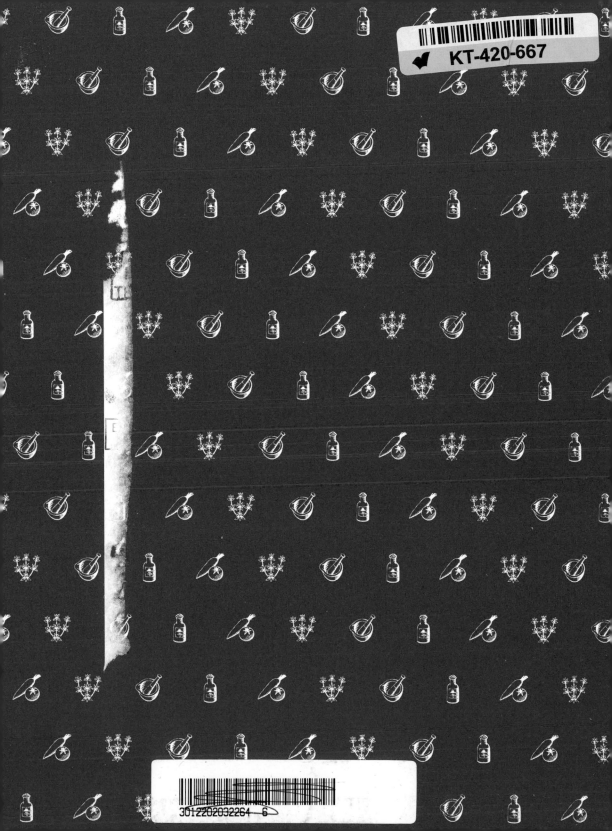

using
Nature's Pharmacy

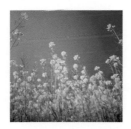

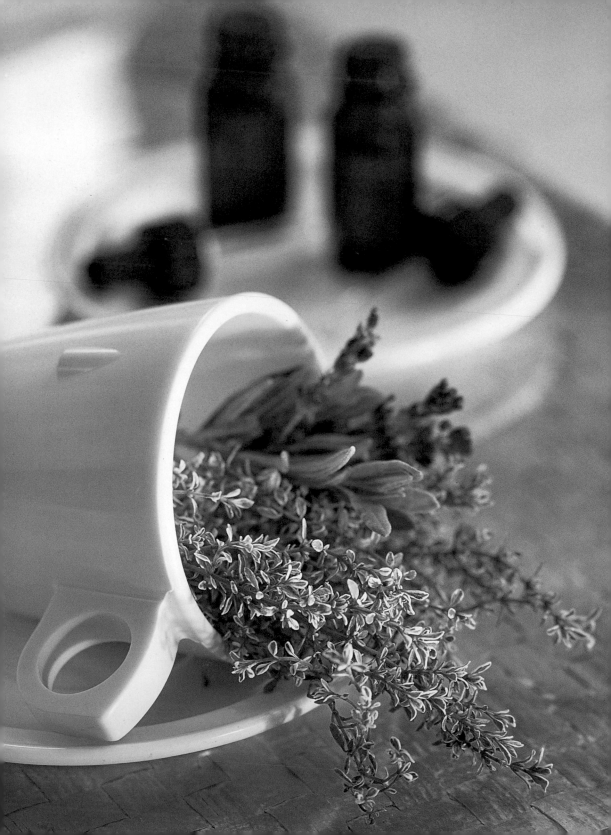

NATURAL HEALING HANDBOOK

using
Nature's Pharmacy

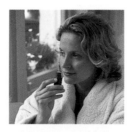

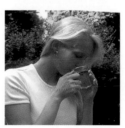

HAYFIELD • HAWKEY • MORNINGSTAR

LORENZ BOOKS

This edition is published by Lorenz Books

Lorenz Books is an imprint of Anness Publishing Ltd
Hermes House, 88–89 Blackfriars Road, London SE1 8HA
tel. 020 7401 2077; fax 020 7633 9499
www.lorenzbooks.com; info@anness.com

© Anness Publishing Ltd 2001, 2002
Published in the USA by Lorenz Books, Anness Publishing Inc., 27 West 20th Street, New York, NY 10011;
fax 212 807 6813

This edition distributed in the UK by Aurum Press Ltd, 25 Bedford Avenue, London WC1B 3AT;
tel. 020 7637 3225; fax 020 7580 2469

This edition distributed in the USA by National Book Network, 4720 Boston Way, Lanham, MD 20706;
tel. 301 459 3366; fax 301 459 1705; www.nbnbooks.com

This edition distributed in Canada by General Publishing, 895 Don Mills Road, 400–402 Park Centre, Toronto,
Ontario M3C 1W3; tel. 416 445 3333; fax 416 445 5991; www.genpub.com

This edition distributed in Australia by Pan Macmillan Australia, Level 18, St Martins Tower, 31 Market St,
Sydney, NSW 2000; tel. 1300 135 113; fax 1300 135 103; email customer.service@macmillan.com.au

This edition distributed in New Zealand by David Bateman Ltd, 30 Tarndale Grove, Off Bush Road, Albany,
Auckland; tel. (09) 415 7664; fax (09) 415 8892

A CIP catalogue record for this book is available from the British Library.

Publisher: Joanna Lorenz
Managing Editor: Helen Sudell
Project Editor: Emma Gray
Additional text by: Stephanie Donaldson, Jessica Houdret and Mark Evans
Designer: Balley Design Associates; Illustrator: Giovanna Pierce
Photographers: Don Last, John Freeman and Michelle Garrett
Production Controller: Claire Rae

Previously published as *Natural Healing*

1 3 5 7 9 10 8 6 4 2

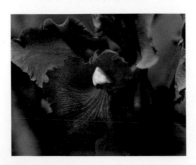

contents

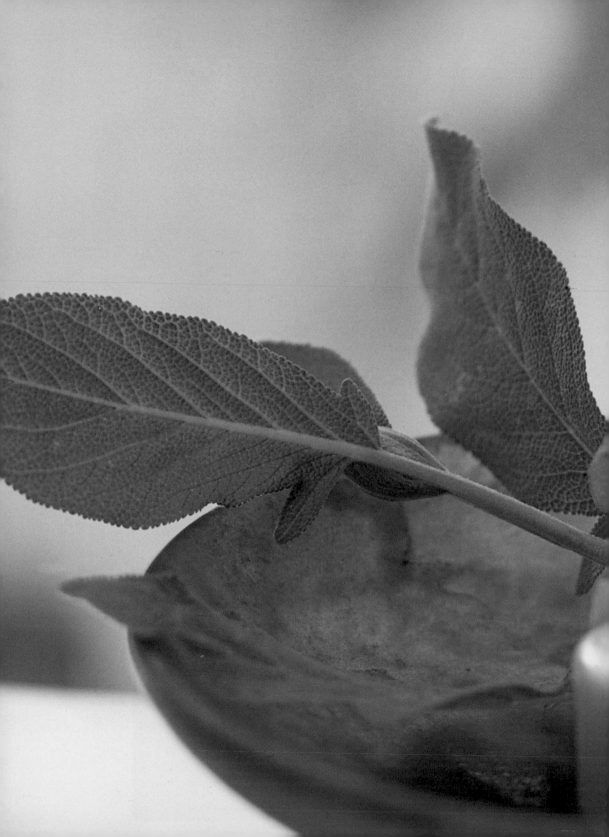

natural natural healing
natural
healing
introduction

One of the key issues today is knowing exactly how to look after yourself, and that does not just mean steering clear of all kinds of excesses that are known to be bad for you, such as coffee, alcohol and stress. It means knowing the many subtle and sophisticated ways in which the body works, which are largely ignored by conventional medicine. Knowing, for example, how the deft use of herbalism can quickly help you to revive after a tiring, difficult day, how using homeopathy can bolster your body's well-being and how the ancient Indian healing technique, Ayurveda, can help you tackle all kinds of illnesses holistically. using diet, colours, gems and crystals.

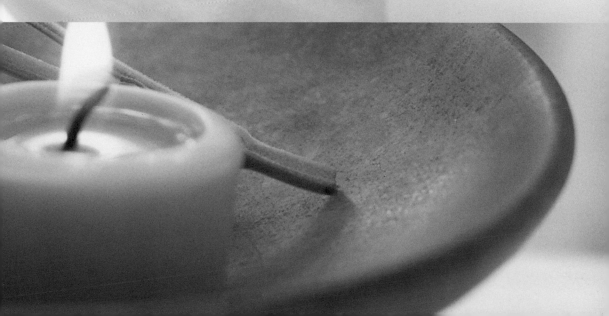

healing naturally

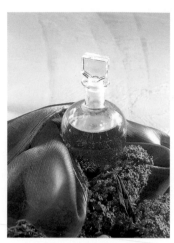

H ealth is the most natural state of being. The root of the word "health" is related not only to "healing" but also to "wholeness", and it is precisely that sense of wholeness and of being in tune – physically, mentally and spiritually – that makes you feel your best. In recent years there has been a massive revival of interest in natural therapies, both in recognition of their tremendous value and as a move away from the impersonal approach and unwelcome side-effects of conventional medicine. Much of this is simply because natural therapists often take more time to get to know the whole person, the whole you, and acknowledge the wider aspects of health. The gentle, natural remedies that they employ have been tried and tested over centuries, and can be effective not just in returning your system to normal when you are ill, but as a means of optimizing your well-being and general state of health.

It is easy to think of medicine only as a crisis treatment for when you are sick, and this is the basis of most ordinary medical practice. Many people neglect their general health until they become ill and then turn to medicine for the cure. Getting the most out

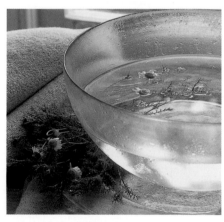

of life means looking after yourself every day and not just trying to cure illness when it arrives. This means boosting your own natural energies to keep yourself in good shape. A healthy body is far less likely to suffer setbacks, and if they do happen it is more likely to cure itself, quickly and completely. Being healthy means being in touch with every part of your being and situation; understanding your strengths and weaknesses and staying true to your character and abilities. One of the strengths of natural therapies is the value they place in early, self-help treatment; in this way the extent of an infection, bacterial or viral, is minimized, and the load that is placed on the immune system is reduced to the barest minimum.

Natural therapies are particularly successful in countering the effects of stress on the body and mind, thus actually helping to reduce the likelihood of illness. Stress is recognized as a major factor affecting health in modern society, but what is little

healing   strengthening
invigorating

understood are the physiological reasons why stress does have such a marked impact on our overall health. Stress re-apportions the supply of blood and nerve energy to different areas, increasing the activity of certain organs and reducing the work of others. In prolonged situations of stress, many functions, vital for everyday health, can be neglected, and over a period of time, the body will begin to suffer and show signs of strain, at which point ill-health will appear, or a weakened condition will worsen. The increasing pace and complexity of modern life, juggling the demands of work and family, places great burdens on the body and it is vital to redress the balance before the strain becomes too great and begins to affect our health. By taking some simple and pleasurable steps to restore

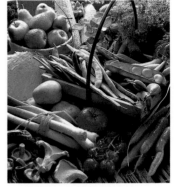

and enhance your own vital energy, you can actively reduce the impact of the worries that you encounter in daily life. Principally, rest is required and attention must be paid to the specific symptoms that you suffer, and this is where this book will offer valuable advice. It is important to try not to spend time worrying about not feeling well, or feeling pressurized, but try and access the nervous energy that comes with stress and use it as a motivational tool to change the things that are affecting your health.

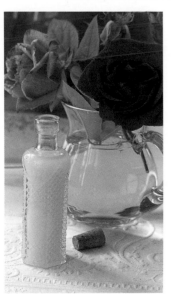

The key to the success of most holistic therapies is that they take into account the mental, emotional and spiritual well-being of a person, as well as the physical aspects of health. Holistic therapies recognize that physical symptoms, such as headaches and stomach upsets, and emotional ones, such as depression, can interweave to create more serious disease.

In order to help reduce the impact of stress on your whole system, you need to find ways both to avoid becoming stressed in the first place, and to release the changes that occur internally. Looking after yourself with a nourishing diet and regular exercise will help you feel better and more able to cope with issues that you really cannot avoid.

The traditions of natural medicine are based on a vast accumulation of practical knowledge. Herbal remedies are almost certainly the most popular and most easily understood

method of self-help treatment. The medicines given are all extracted from plants, and as with many other complementary treatments they may also be combined with other general health advice. Herbalism is excellent for minor complaints and such problems as anxiety, indigestion and hangovers; the problems can be simply and easily treated using herbal cures that are easy to make. Infusions, which are rather like herb teas, are a delicious and safe way to take medicinal herbs. Herbs may also be taken as tinctures or syrups. Scented herbal baths are a real pleasure and remarkably effective for treating certain complaints. Herbal remedies will alleviate many common

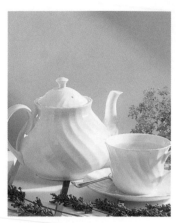

symptoms, and there are numerous simple herbal recipes in this book that can be used.

Illnesses can also be treated with homeopathic remedies which you can administer yourself. Homeopathy was discovered in the 18th century by Samuel Hahnemann who began the experiments that led to the development and principles of the modern therapy. In homeopathy, symptoms are seen not as the negative effects of illness, but as the attempts of the individual to resist disease. Hence a remedy that produces the symptoms of a particular illness in a healthy person is administered in minute doses to a person with those symptoms. Homeopaths describe this as treating "like with like". Since the remedies are given in such minute doses, it is surmised that they

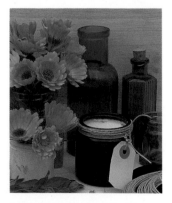

are acting not on the physical body, but on the surrounding energies of the body. This encourages and supports the body's own self-healing mechanisms, enabling it to combat the disease effectively and in a natural manner that is controlled by the body itself.

Traditional healing therapies have evolved in most cultures in the East and in the West. The ancient Indian system of Ayurveda is thought to be one of the oldest healing disciplines in the world. Like much of Eastern ideology, it involves energy: it views all parts of the human body as being interconnected and infused with vital forces, which are constantly revitalizing themselves. The body is not just regarded as an empty vessel into which you pour the

herbalism
homeopathy
ayurveda

wholeness gentleness energizing invigorating soothing healing

remedies prescribed by conventional medicine when something goes wrong. Ayurvedic medicine is just one facet of a complete Ayurvedic philosophy and way of life. It recognizes that most people can be characterized into various basic categories, and it offers dietary and exercise regimes suited to each of these. You can draw on the ancient principles of Ayurveda to help balance your energies by following a lifestyle suited to your particular character and body type. At the same time, recognizing the type of person you are will enhance your self awareness and help you to appreciate how your lifestyle is impinging and perhaps detracting from your current state of health and well-being. Ayurveda is the origin of many branches of complementary therapies today and uses colour infusions and herbal remedies, as well as crystal-healing, aromatherapy and massage, to help return the body to health. It truly is an all-round healing therapy that is very effective and appeals to a great many people.

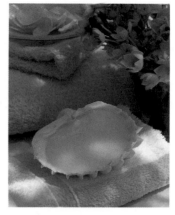

All three natural therapies described here, herbalism, homeopathy and ayurveda, take time to examine the various symptoms of a person's illness and usually also offer preventative advice for the future. Perhaps it is this overall evaluation of the illness and then relating it to the whole person, combined with the self-help advice, that sets apart many complementary therapies from conventional medical practices. There is no doubt that it is refreshing to take back some of the responsibility for our own health, and

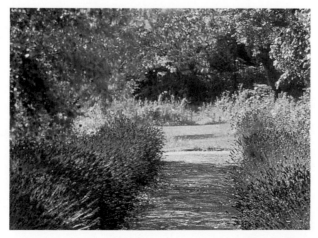

encouraging to know that we can work with our own bodies and with nature by using the materials they have to offer to keep us well. Although there are some uncontrollable external factors that affect our health, armed with a little knowledge of complementary medicine, we can enjoy vastly improved health, enabling us to live and enjoy our lives to the full.

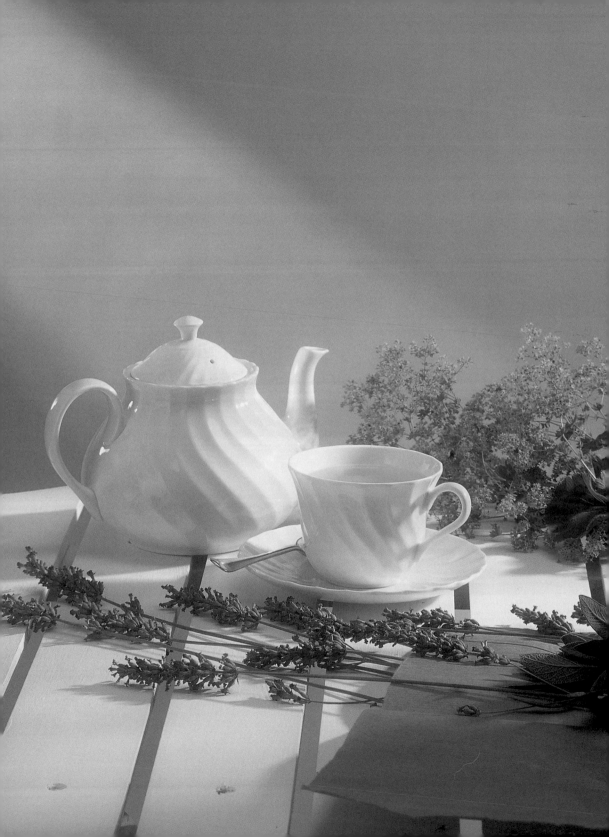

herbalism
herbalism

herbalism

All over the world, people have used plants not only as food but also as medicines. Traditional knowledge of herbal remedies used to be passed from generation to generation, but nowadays this is rare.

Fortunately, the countryside still produces wonderful herbs and many can be grown in the garden. Getting to know the plants growing around you can be a relaxing pleasure in itself. If you learn about their various properties, you can use them to help you feel more healthy and better able to cope with everyday problems. Very simple remedies can easily be made from dried or fresh herbs, and substituting an excellent herb tea for stimulating drinks such as tea, coffee and cola will help you to relax and reduce your tension levels.

Herbs, like people, are complex and variable organic structures. Each plant contains many different constituents which together give a unique taste and range of actions. Particularly active constituents have been isolated and copied by pharmacists to produce medicines such as aspirin. However, using the whole plant has a much more subtle effect, and generates far fewer side effects. Herbalists therefore prefer to use the whole plant to treat the whole person. We are all unique and react to life in different ways; just as we all have special preferences for various foods, each of us responds best to particular herbs.

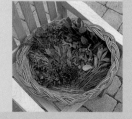

the nervous system
It is easily overlooked, but the nervous system is like the key component in a highly complex computer. It regulates and fine tunes, analyses information and decides on the best course of action; it is an extremely sophisticated kind of mechanism. That is why looking after the nervous system is one of the most important things you can do. Here are some excellent ways of making sure that you relax and keep feeling well.

The Effects of Stress

The involuntary or autonomic nervous system has two divisions. The sympathetic part prepares you for action and initiates the "fight or flight" response. The parasympathetic system is responsible for the body's "housekeeping", ensuring good digestion, assimilation of nutrients, detoxification and elimination of waste products. The sympathetic system allows you to respond to any stimulation, making the heart and lungs more active when necessary and suppressing natural processes such as digestion.

   All life follows a natural rhythm, with periods of activity followed by periods of rest. This is as it should be. Too much stimulation, or an over-reaction to stimulation, leads to stress. If you are subjected to excess stimulation, sympathetic activities become dominant or habitual and may reach a state of exhaustion, reducing your ability to react and cope appropriately with new stresses. This can cause forgetfulness, panic, exhaustion or increased vulnerability to infection. At the same time, reduced parasympathetic activity can cause all sorts of digestive and nutritional debilities as well as poor elimination, which in turn can result in problems with the skin, muscles or joints.

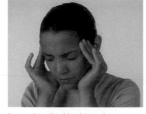

Lavender oil rubbed into the temples will encourage relaxation, and gradually ease a headache.

Helpful Herbs

The nervous system co-ordinates all the highly complex activities that manage to keep us functioning efficiently and well. They help us rapidly, unconsciously adjust to all kinds of constantly changing stimuli. The following pages clearly describe some of the highly valuable, beautiful plants growing right across the world which, among their many properties, help give back-up and support to the nervous system. Herbalists have named these very important plants, the nervines.

Choosing the Right Remedies

Like all herbs, nervines have a wide range of actions. It is important that you choose the one that applies to your own symptoms of stress, and to which you feel naturally drawn. Knowing, growing, harvesting and drying herbs (which is quite easily done) will help you to appreciate them much more. You may well discover that a symptom that is particularly troubling can in fact be treated by several different remedies.

Simply meandering down paths of richly scented lavender can quickly help to raise the spirits.

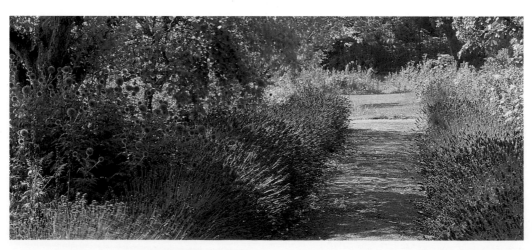

Nervous Tonics

These plants are used to aid recovery from stress and are particularly useful when we feel in any way debilitated and exhausted after an illness, prolonged pressure or even a trauma. They will improve the health and functioning of nervous tissue by invigorating and restoring it.

Some act as gentle stimulants while others are in fact slightly more sedating. Your choice will depend on whether nervous debility makes you hyperactive (in which case choose relaxing nervines) or restless, depressed and tired (in which case you must choose stimulating nervines).

Stimulating Tonics:

- Mugwort (Artemisia vulgaris)
- Wild Oats (Avena sativa)
- St John's Wort (Hypericum perforatum)
- Sage (Salvia officinalis)
- Damiana (Turnera diffusa)

Relaxing Tonics:

- Wood Betony (Stachys betonica)
- Skullcap (Scutellaria lateriflora)
- Vervain (Verbena officinalis)

Stimulants

Some plants, such as coffee and tea, stimulate our nervous system without nourishing it. Since such over-stimulation is exhausting, additional herbal stimulants are rarely used. But there is a place for gently stimulating nervines. For example, Mugwort is beneficial during convalescence and Rosemary, by helping stimulate blood flow to the head, is used to tackle and reduce tension headaches.

- Rosemary (Rosmarinus officinalis)

Relaxants and Sedatives

You can use relaxing nervines to calm yourself down and prevent over-stimulation. All these valuable herbs will help encourage rest and sleep. In any event some, like the Passion Flower and Lime Blossom, are excellent garden plants and help create a marvellous soothing atmosphere; a garden made for quietly walking round, inhaling the excellent scents, filled with a wide range of colours.

- Lady's Mantle (Alchemilla xanthochlora)
- Pasque Flower (Anemone pulsatilla)
- Chamomile (Chamaemelum nobile and Chamomilla recutita)
- Californian Poppy (Eschscholtzia californica)
- Hops (Humulus lupulus)
- Lavender (Lavandula spp.)
- Motherwort (Leonurus cardiaca)
- Lemon Balm (Melissa officinalis)
- Peppermint (Mentha piperita)
- Marjoram (Origanum vulgare)
- Passion Flower (Passiflora incarnata)
- Lime Blossom (Tilia x europaea)
- Cramp Bark (Viburnum opulus)
- Valerian (Valeriana officinalis)

Adaptogens

- Siberian Ginseng (Eleutheroccocus senticosus)
- Korean Ginseng (Panax spp.)

Other useful Herbs

- Borage (Borage officinalis)
- Licorice (Glycyrrhiza glabra)
- Evening Primrose (Oenothera biennis)
- Chaste Tree (Vitex agnus-castus)

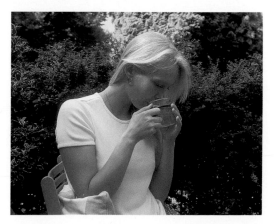

Taking Herbal Preparations

Like other medicines, herbal remedies must be taken at the appropriate time and in a suitable manner tailored to the individual. For example, in cases of pregnancy, no strong herbal teas should be taken during the first trimester, even if they would otherwise relieve stress because the body is in too sensitive a state. Likewise, young children, whose bodies are also very labile, should not take Peppermint or Sage tea, they may suffer an adverse reaction. It is commonsense to avoid ready-made herbal mixes that contain sugar, the sugar will only create an additional burden for the body, reducing its ability to cope. Where it is possible, the cause of the stress should be removed, and everything done to support the person at this time.

Herbal teas are easily made in a wide range of flavours. They are a gentle and simple way to soothe both body and mind.

the herb garden
Herb gardens are easy to make and quickly stocked. Get a catalogue from a specialist seed supplier and you will probably find that they have eight or so different kinds of Basil from Europe and the Far East, with herbs like Coriander and Cumin. Growing them is incredibly easy. In most cases, pick regularly to encourage plenty of fresh, new tasty shoots. You will quickly see the benefits in the kitchen and your health.

PLANTING HERBS
You do not need very much space to grow herbs: a small border, or even a collection of containers, will provide a perfectly good supply. But if you do have the room, a large herb garden offers the chance to try fun designs like a circle of triangular beds pointing in to a focal point such as a small statue or painted urn.

Soil and Site
Most herbs are undemanding and quick to grow. They are essentially wild plants, and do not require rich, highly cultivated soil. Many of the most useful herbs, such as Sage, Thyme, Rosemary and Lavender, are natives of southern Europe and will not survive heavy clay soils or water-logged conditions. Many moisture-loving plants, such as Lemon Balm, Mint and Valerian, will grow happily in a light soil, though not in conditions of total drought. A sunny, sheltered position protected from strong biting winds will suit all the plants, though some, such as the more tender Lemon Verbena and Bay, will need protecting in bad winters.

Design
A formal layout of small beds dissected by paths provides a satisfying framework for the lax, untidy growth of many herbs. It also makes sure that you can easily tend and pick when necessary. A single species to each bed can look highly effective, evoking the magical, atmospheric style of medieval herb gardens. In contrast, an informal cottage garden provides plenty of scope for imaginative, exuberant planting with herbs cleverly mixed in with flowers. Raised beds or a lively collection of attractive containers make easy-to-control, self-contained areas.

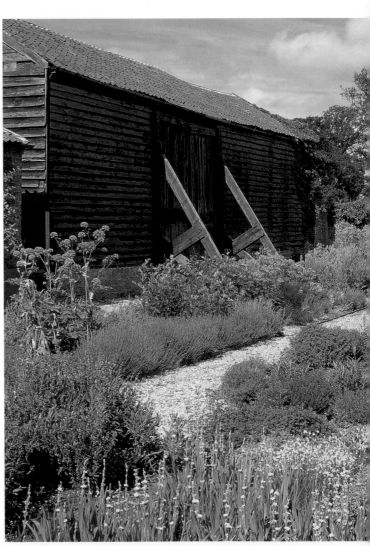

A perfect example of a well-tended herb garden, with symmetrical beds and wide paths for easy access. The plants thrive in this warm, sheltered corner of the garden.

EXPERIENCING HERBS

Identifying, growing and harvesting herbs can be a marvellous, healing experience itself. Handling herbs brings you closer to nature and increases your appreciation of the vitality of plants.

Growing

The quickest way to acquire herbs that will help you stay healthy is to grow them yourself. You can easily grow most from seed. This means that you will be sure what they are, and that they will have been grown safely and organically, without the use of any chemical sprays. Most of the herbs used in the remedies on the following pages will grow extremely well in temperate climates. In fact many are often regarded as weeds, and actually thrive on patches of spare ground despite getting no care and attention whatsoever.

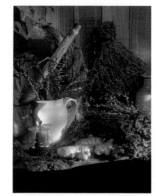

Many of the culinary herbs we use today were distributed throughout Europe by the Roman army.

Gathering

The aerial parts of herbs (the flowers, stems and leaves) should be gathered for use or for drying when the plants are in bud and totally dry. That means early morning when the sun has dried the dew. Roots should be dug in the autumn, cleaned and roughly chopped into very small pieces.

If you harvest from the wild, make quite sure that you have identified the plant correctly (use a good wild flower book) and that it has not been polluted by fertilizers, pesticides or car fumes. Never pick so much that you reduce next year's growth.

Drying

Spread out your herbs on a rack to dry naturally in an airy position, out of direct sunlight. Alternatively, tie them in loose bundles and hang them from a beam, or dry them in an oven at a very low heat.

Storing

Always make sure that you store dried herbs in airtight containers, kept well away from the light, and do not forget to label and date them. They will keep for up to six months, but the sooner they are used the better and fresher the flavour. (When they are kept for too long they look dull and taste of sawdust.) If you are in any way worried about over-drying your herbs, try storing them in a freezer instead. This is a particularly good technique for herbs such as Lemon Balm and Parsley, which quickly lose their flavour when they are dried.

Buying

Many shops stock dried herbs. Buy these only if they seem fresh – they should be brightly coloured and strongly aromatic.

Some herbal remedies are now readily available over the counter in the form of capsules, tablets or tinctures. These are usually of good quality. Choose the simpler ones that tell you exactly the type and quantity of herb involved.

Lime Blossom is abundant for easy picking in both the countryside and urban areas during early summer.

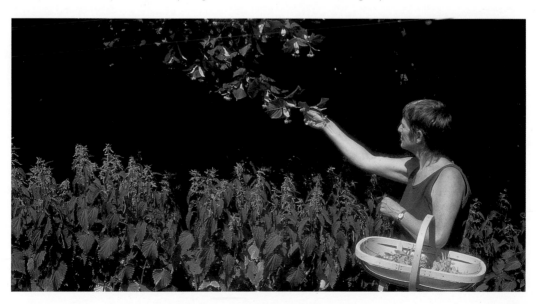

herbal preparations

Herbs are multi-talented. They can be used in the kitchen, fresh or dried, and to tackle a wide range of ailments from hyperactivity to insomnia. They even provide a refreshing tonic when you are feeling down-and-out. In fact, you can take herbal remedies internally as teas, decoctions and tinctures, or applied externally as soothing, relaxing oils and conditioners. Best of all, they guarantee gorgeous perfumes.

MAKING TEAS

Herbal teas are also called infusions or tisanes. They are a simple and delicious way of extracting the goodness and flavour from the aerial parts of herbs. You can use either fresh or dried herbs to make such teas; note you need to use twice as much fresh plant material as dried. If you find the taste of some herb teas rather bitter, then try sweetening them with a little honey. Alternatively, try adding extra flavour by stirring the tea with a Licorice stick, or adding ginger.

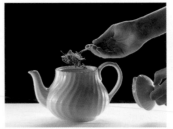

1 Put your herb(s) into a pot. Standard-strength tea is made with 1 tsp dried or 2 tsp fresh herbs to 1 cup of water.

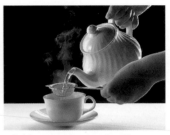

2 Strain and drink as required. Teas can be drunk cold as well as hot. Cold teas are thoroughly invigorating.

MAKING DECOCTIONS

Infusing in boiling water is not enough to extract the constituents from roots or bark. This much tougher, harder, inflexible plant material needs to be broken up into far smaller pieces by chopping or crushing with a sharp knife.

Next, place every tiny scrap of this rough-cut material into a stainless steel, glass or enamelled pan, but absolutely not aluminium. Fill up with cold water, and gradually bring to the boil. Finally cover and simmer for about 15 minutes. The resulting liquid is what is called a decoction. Strain it and flavour, if necessary, and drink while it is still warm.

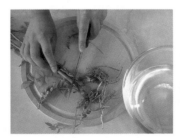

1 Harvest root and bark in the colder months. Trim the aerial parts of the plant away from the root.

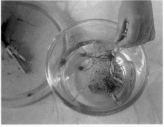

2 Wash the roots thoroughly in cold water, ensuring they are perfectly clean, then chop into small pieces.

Nervine Decoctions

- Cramp Bark
- Licorice
- Valerian

Avoid using Licorice if you suffer from high blood pressure.

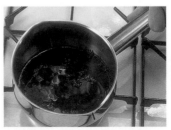

3 Fill a pan with cold water and add 1 tsp of the chopped herb per cup. Boil and simmer for 10–15 minutes.

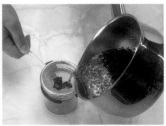

4 Strain and cool before drinking. Decoctions can be kept for 24 hours in the fridge. Drink reheated or cold.

MAKING TINCTURES

Sometimes it is more convenient to take a spoonful of medicine than make a tea or decoction. Tinctures are made by steeping herbs in a mixture of alcohol and water. The alcohol extracts the medicinal constituents, and it also acts as an excellent preservative.

Herb syrups make good remedies for giving to children. They also improve the taste of herbs that might be bitter, such as Motherwort and Vervain.

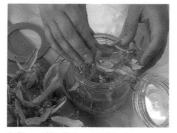

I Place 100 g/3½ oz dried herbs or 300g/11 oz fresh herbs in a jar.

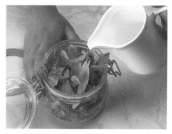

2 Add 250ml/8fl oz/1 cup vodka and 250ml/8fl oz/1 cup water.

Making Syrups

I Place 500g/1¼lb sugar/honey in a pan; add 1 litre/1¾ pints/4 cups water.
2 Heat gently, stirring to dissolve.
3 Add 150g/5oz plant material and heat gently for 5 minutes.
4 Turn off the heat; steep overnight.
5 Strain and store in an airtight container for future use. Since the sugar acts as a preservative, a herb syrup will keep for 18 months.

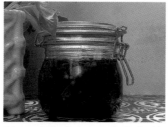

3 Leave the herbs to steep in the liquid for a month, preferably on a sunny windowsill. Gently shake the jar daily.

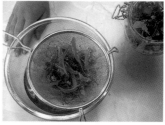

4 Strain and store the tincture in a dark glass bottle where it will keep well for approximately 18 months.

COLD INFUSED OILS

Herbal oils are suitable for external use when having a massage, or as bath oils or hair and skin conditioners. Cold infused oils are quite simple to prepare. Macerate freshly cut herbs in vegetable oil for up to two weeks, but no more. Give the jar a daily shake. Finally drain off the oil, and squeeze the excess liquid out of the herbs. You will find that chamomile invariably gives excellent results.

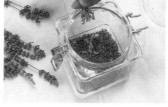

I Fill a glass storage jar with the flowers or leaves of your chosen dried herb.

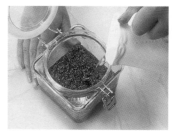

2 Pour in a vegetable oil to cover the herbs; try sunflower or grape seed oil.

Herb Oil Infusions

- Chamomile
- Lavender
- Marjoram
- Rosemary
- St John's Wort

Do not put St John's Wort oil on the skin before going into bright sunshine for fear of an adverse reaction.

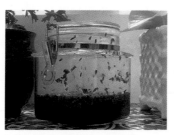

3 Stand the jar for two weeks on a windowsill to steep. Shake daily.

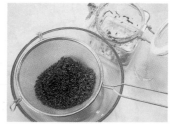

4 Strain. For a stronger infusion, renew the herbs in the oil every two weeks.

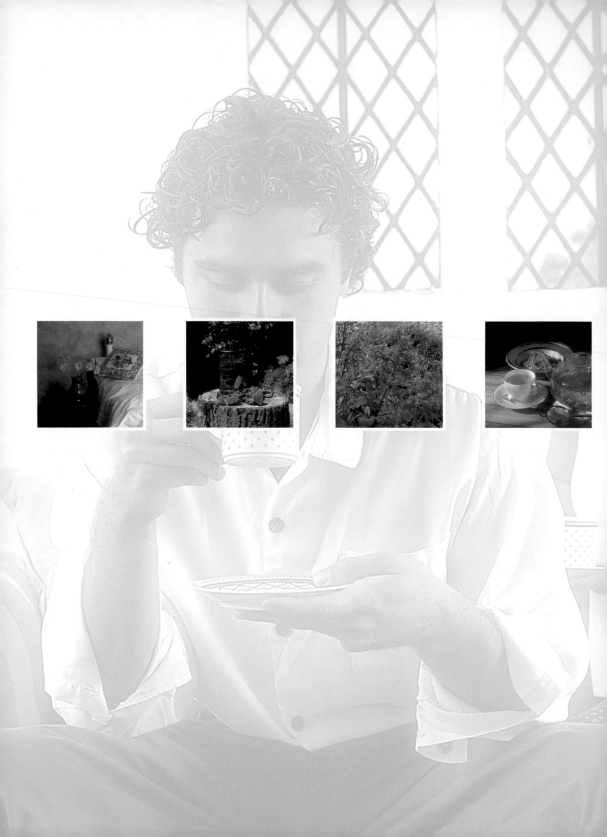

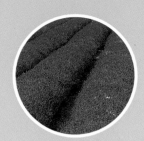

herbal recipes
herbal recipes

herbal recipes

In today's high-tech, high-speed world it is virtually impossible not to encounter stress, and stress at even alarmingly high levels. It can strike going to work when you get stuck in a gridlock traffic jam, at work with faxes, e-mails and meetings, and when you get back home and suddenly have to cope with meals and children. In fact, many people find that getting quality, quiet time for themselves is becoming increasingly difficult, if not impossible. But while you cannot always avoid stress, there are plenty of things you can do to help yourself cope better when life suddenly presents a barrage of testing, difficult challenges.

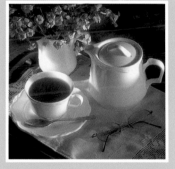

A good, healthy diet really does make a significant difference. It is therefore absolutely essential that you eat proper, healthy meals packed with vitamin-rich fruit and vegetables, and totally avoid artificial additives. If you miss these extra flavours, you will find that you get a far greater range using fresh or dried herbs, and of course they offer plenty of extra goodness.

Also, try as hard as you can to reduce your intake of such stimulants as tea, coffee, alcohol and cola. Instead, drink plenty of water and invigorating herbal teas. All kinds of flavours are becoming increasingly available. You simply choose what you like, and that can include Anise, Chamomile, Lemon Verbena, Lime Blossom, Mint, and Sage. They are all incredibly refreshing. Even better, you can grow these herbs in pots or in the garden, where you know they have been organically raised.

Exercise is equally important for all kinds of reasons. It dispels excess adrenaline and improves relaxation and sleep. Swimming prevents your joints from becoming stiff and gives the body a marvellous feeling of freedom. Exercise also tones up your muscles, keeps you in shape, and helps shed excess weight. In short, it keeps you feeling alert, well and able.

One of the biggest problems of stress is that it can all too easily disrupt your appetite and your ability to rest. In turn, such disruption makes you even less able to cope with any setbacks and problems. You get pulled into a depressing, downward spiral. One of the best ways to break out of this pattern is to use herbal remedies to improve your digestion, to help you relax, and to improve your adaptability.

The recipes that follow are designed to help you through difficult times. As long as you do not exceed the doses stated, and are sure that you are using the right plant, it is safe to experiment with these suggestions. But do seek professional help if a problem persists.

key stress symptoms

While some degree of stress is an inevitable part of modern life, there are fortunately several significant ways of tackling it. They should help make sure that your day is not ruined by a tense neck or a nervous stomach. In fact some ways, such as using using excellent massage oils, are so incredibly relaxing, refreshing and enjoyable that they could well become part of your daily routine.

CALMING ANXIETY

Everyone knows exactly what it feels like to be excited, but inappropriate or excessive excitement, often combined with frustration, creates anxiety. In this state, the body produces too much adrenaline. It is primed for "fight or flight" but neither is possible. The heart races, muscles tense and the chest expands. Anxiety can cause many symptoms, including palpitations, sweating, irritability and sleeplessness. In these situations, Rescue Remedy, which is bought ready-made, is useful.

Two drops of Rescue Remedy on the tongue can help prevent a panic attack, and give you ease of mind.

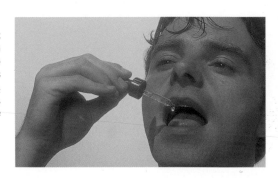

RELAXING TENSE MUSCLES

Muscles can tense as a result of anxiety which often causes slightly raised shoulders or contracted back muscles. The effort of maintaining your muscles in this semi-contracted state is tiring, possibly causing spasms and bad postural habits. The neck stiffens and the back may ache. Tight neck muscles can also hinder blood flowing to the head, creating tension headaches. Moving frequently will release the muscles. Rotate your head or stand and stretch, and take breaks from working or driving. Gently massaging the neck with oil can help.

Tension can build up in the neck and shoulders, causing stiffness.

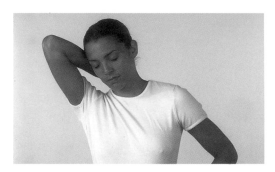

Cold Infused Oil of Lavender

Fill a glass jar with lavender heads and cover with clear vegetable oil. Allow to steep on a windowsill, shaking the jar every day. Strain and bottle.

The oil can be used for massaging into a stiff neck or back. It can also be added to the bath to keep your skin soft and perfumed, while also encouraging relaxation.

Lavender is an extremely talented herb. It has traditionally been used as a sedative helping combat anxiety and tension. A few drops of infused oil added to your favourite massage oil will also help relax your over-tense muscles. Similar oils can be made from Marjoram (which is anti-spasmodic) and Rosemary.

Herbal Remedies

To help your nervous system readjust and adapt, consider the value of:
- Skullcap
- St John's Wort
- Vervain
- Wild Oats
- Wood Betony

Choose whichever one suits you best and combine it with a specific remedy for the symptom that is causing you most problems.
- To ease palpitations: Motherwort or Passion Flower.
- To reduce sweating: Motherwort or Valerian.
- To help you sleep: Passion Flower.

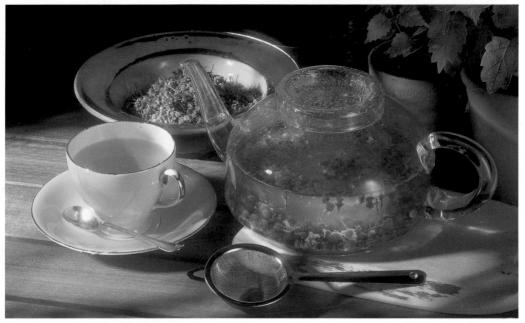

Chamomile tea makes an ideal after-dinner drink.

DIGESTIVES

Many people suffer from digestive upsets when they are stressed. This is because the "fight or flight" activity of the sympathetic nervous system tends to suppress digestive processes. The result may be indigestion, loss of appetite, wind, diarrhoea or even an irritable bowel.

The three recipes below have all been specially designed to help relax the nervous system, encouraging parasympathetic activity and reducing any signs of spasm in the gut.

To Calm Butterflies

Nervous stomachs can be quickly settled by Chamomile, Hops and Lemon Balm combined in a tea, or simply select the best combination for you. Lemon Balm and Chamomile can be taken as frequently as you like.

Put I tsp each Lemon Balm, dried Chamomile flowers and Peppermint into a small tea pot or cafetière. Fill with boiling water and allow to steep for at least 10 minutes. Strain and drink at least three times a day or after meals.

Herbal Remedies	
• Chamomile	• Hops
• Cramp Bark	• Lemon Balm
• Cumin	• Licorice
• Fennel, Caraway, Dill	• Peppermint

To Relieve Wind and Colic

In a small saucepan, boil I tsp each Fennel seeds and Cramp Bark with about 300ml/½ pint/1¼ cups water. Add I tsp dried Peppermint. Allow to steep for 10 minutes. Strain and drink.

To Ease Constipation

Make a decoction of Cramp Bark and Fennel as above, but add I tsp Licorice root. If the constipation is proving to be an unpleasant, recurrent condition, I tsp Linseeds added daily to your breakfast cereal can be very helpful.

The same amount can also be soaked in hot water for about two hours, and drunk before going to bed and again, if necessary, early the next morning when you wake. If the problem is not eased or solved then it is important that you consult your doctor at the first opportunity. Generally, the best way to avoid an attack of constipation is to make sure that you are regularly having a balanced, healthy diet which includes plenty of fresh fruit, vegetables and roughage on a daily basis.

Contraindications

Some herbs should only be used at certain times and not if you are suffering certain other symptoms. For example, since Hops are a sedative, they should only be taken at night, and are not suitable if you are depressed or lacking in sexual energy. Likewise, Licorice should be avoided if you have high blood pressure or oedema. Always consult a medical doctor if in any doubt.

revitalizing recipes

You do not have to be so ill that you are completely confined to bed to take some of the excellent revitalizing herbal remedies now available. Many are purpose designed as a refreshing pick-me-up or tonic to get you through testing emotional and physical times – the bad, dark days – when the mind and body might otherwise become tired and sluggish. Such recipes are nature's way of keeping you healthy.

NERVOUS EXHAUSTION

It is much more likely that you will get ill or depressed after or during a long period of hard work, or from a whole battery of emotional demands. This can easily happen to teachers, for example, at the end of term, or to those who have to care for disabled or sick relations on a long-term basis. You will find that herbal remedies help to give your nervous system plenty of vital support at such testing, difficult times. To make a revitalizing tea, mix equal portions of all the dried herbs listed. Put 3–4 tsp of the mixture into a pot with a lid. Add 600ml/1 pint/2½ cups boiling water. Steep for 10 minutes, strain, and drink 3–4 cups a day.

Herbal Remedies	
• Borage	• St John's Wort
• Licorice	• Wild Oats
• Skullcap	• Wood Betony

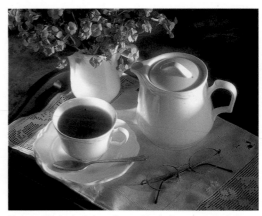

Make a relaxing herbal tea from a blend of supportive herbs whenever you are feeling exhausted and too tired to cope.

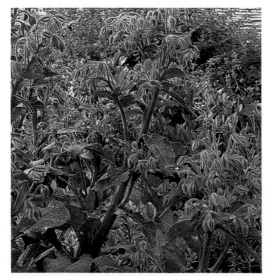

Borage, like Licorice, restores the adrenal glands.

TONICS FOR CONVALESCENCE

Remember that even if your symptoms have gone, your body needs time to recover after an illness. A tonic is extremely useful. Wild Oats and St John's Wort support the nervous system, Vervain promotes relaxation and digestion, and Licorice restores the adrenal glands. Vitamin C supplements should be continued for several weeks after an illness. Alfalfa sprouts are also high in vitamins and minerals. Also note that rest is very important.

Tonic Tea

Put ½ tsp of each of one of the dried herbs listed below into a small pot. Add boiling water. Flavour with Peppermint to taste. (Avoid Licorice if you suffer from high blood pressure or oedema.) Allow to steep for 10 minutes. Strain. Drink three or four cups, warm, each day for at least three weeks.

Herbal Remedies	
• Borage	• Vervain
• Licorice	• Wild Oats
• St John's Wort	

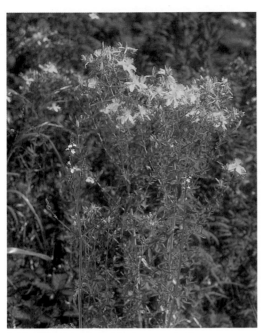

St John's Wort thrives in a bright, open sunny position.

RELIEVING WINTER BLUES

The old herbalists thought that the appearance of a plant held a clue to its healing action. For instance, Pilewort (Lesser Celandine) has roots that resemble haemorrhoids, and it does indeed make an effective ointment for piles. The flowers of St John's Wort resemble nothing so much as the sun. The plant thrives in sunlight and is known to have anti-depressant effects. There is no better herb than this to take if you are depressed in the winter, when sunlight is in short supply.

Wild Oats also help by strengthening the nervous system and keeping you warm. Rosemary, an evergreen plant, will improve circulation to the head and keep the mind clear. Also, Ginseng capsules can be taken for a month in the early autumn to help you adapt to the difficult transition between seasons.

Winter Brightener

Combine 2 tsp dried St John's Wort with 1 tsp dried Rosemary. Add 250ml/8fl oz/1 cup boiling water. Allow to steep for 10 minutes and then strain. One cup alone is not enough. Drink three times a day throughout the winter.

Herbal Remedies	
• Ginseng	• St John's Wort
• Rosemary	• Wild Oats

LIFTING DEPRESSION

Depression is a very good illustration of the close connection that exists between the body and mind: physical and emotional energy are both depleted when you are in a depressed state. Both will benefit from a healthy diet that includes plenty of raw, vital foods, nuts, seeds and B vitamins. A multi-vitamin and mineral supplement is an effective kick-start that will give you an excellent lift. But do not undermine its effect by indulging in stimulants, such as caffeine, because they tend to exhaust both the body and mind.

The refreshing, restorative tea described below is a marvellous, tasty way of restoring the health of your nervous system. It has a slight, barely noticeable, stimulating effect.

Restorative Tea

Mix equal parts of each of the dried herbs listed in the box below. Put 2 tsp of the mixture into a pot. Add 600ml/1 pint/2½ cups boiling water. Allow to steep for 10 minutes and then strain. Drink one cup of this excellent tea three times a day.

Herbal Remedies	
• Damiana	• Wild Oats
• St John's Wort	

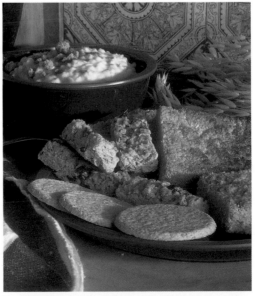

There are many tasty ways of incorporating the goodness of Oats in your diet, including home-made snacks such as biscuits.

headache and night-time remedies

From time to time everyone suffers from headaches and bad sleepless nights. Occasional attacks are just about bearable, but when they become a regular feature and interrupt your life, especially your sex life, it is clearly time to act. All these herbal solutions, ranging from baths and teas to massages, have one aim: to give you back your healthy life as quickly as possible.

RELIEVING TENSION HEADACHES

Headaches are a common symptom of stress. Often they are caused by tension in the neck and upper back muscles. This can prevent adequate blood supply to the head and thus lead to pain. Both massage and exercise can ease this kind of headache.

Scented Baths

Pour a few drops of essential oil or infused oil into a hot bath, lie back and relax. Better, tie a bunch of herbs under the hot tap as you fill the bath. Rub two drops of essential oil of Lavender mixed with 1 tsp water on the head when stressed.

Soothing Tea

Put 1 tsp dried Wood Betony and ½ tsp dried Lavender or Rosemary into a cup. Top up with boiling water and leave for 10 minutes, before straining and drinking. Repeat hourly.

Herbal remedies	
• Lavender	• Rosemary

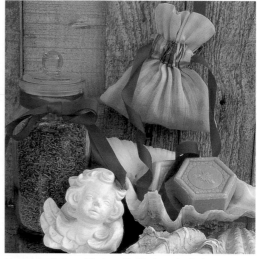

Hang a muslin bag of fresh or dried herbs under the hot tap.

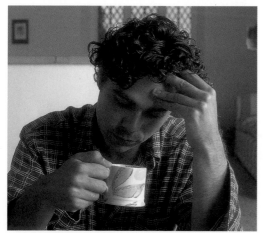

Help yourself beat a hangover by taking a herbal remedy.

HANGOVER REMEDIES

Most people know what a hangover feels like – a combination of headache, nausea, fuzzy head and depression. Most of these symptoms are connected with the liver being overloaded. Bitter herbs stimulate the liver and speed up its ability to detoxify. Vervain is bitter and Lavender aids digestion; both herbs also lift the spirits. If you have a hangover it is also advisable to drink plenty of water and take extra vitamin C.

Morning-After Tea

Put 1 tsp dried Vervain and ½ tsp Lavender flowers into a pot. Add 600ml/1 pint/2½ cups boiling water and cover to keep in the volatile oils. Steep for 10 minutes. Strain and sweeten with a little honey. Sip through the day until you start to feel better.

Herbal Remedies	
• Lavender	• Vervain

REVITALIZING THE LIBIDO

Depression or anxiety can all too easily hinder and interrupt your sex life. This may be because your energy is too low, or it may in fact be connected with a hormone imbalance. Damiana stimulates both the nervous and hormonal systems, and it has vital constituents which convert to hormones in the body. Vervain is good at releasing tension and stress, and it was traditionally used as an aphrodisiac. Wild Oats and Ginger root are both considered stimulating too.

Energizing Tea

Put 1 tsp dried Damiana and 1 tsp dried Vervain into a pot. Add 600ml/1 pint/2½ cups of boiling water. Leave to steep for 10 minutes. Strain and flavour with Licorice, Ginger or honey, as you prefer. Drink two cups a day.

Herbal Remedies	
• Damiana	• Vervain
• Ginger	• Wild Oats

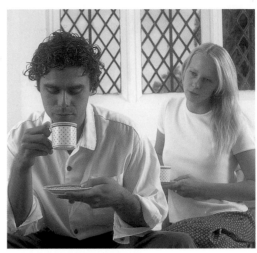

Teas or decoctions made with the right herbs can help restore energy of all kinds, including sexual energy.

ENHANCING SLEEP

There are many different types of insomnia, and the causes are varied. If you really cannot sleep then it is best to experiment with the remedies below to find the one herb or combination of herbs that suits you best. If the problem is long term and you have not been sleeping well for a period of time, then take a nervous system tonic to improve your well being.

In the evenings, drink teas that have been made from relaxing herbs. Lavender oil in a hot bath before bed and on the pillow will also help. You could even try using a Hop pillow. Furthermore, it is important to give yourself plenty of time at the end of the day to relax and wind down. Exercise, meditation and yoga are all good at helping you fall asleep.

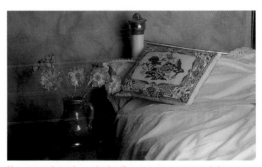

You can make or buy a herb pillow to encourage sound sleep.

Sleepy Tea

Put 1 tsp each dried Chamomile, Vervain and Lemon Balm into a pot. Add about 600ml/1 pint/2½ cups boiling water. Leave to steep for 10 minutes. Strain and drink one cup after supper. Warm the rest and drink before going to bed.

If you continue to have problems sleeping, add a decoction of 1 tsp Valerian root or ½ tsp dried Hops or Californian Poppy to this blend of herbs.

Herbal Remedies	
• Californian Poppy	• Passion Flower
• Chamomile	• Valerian
• Hops	• Vervain
• Lemon Balm	

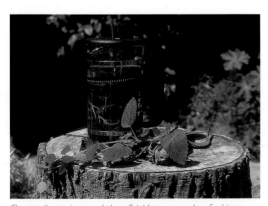

Chamomile tea is not only beneficial but extremely refreshing.

herbal facials

The skin is all too sensitive to poor health and is easily damaged, not in dramatic ways but in gradual, subtle ways that can easily make it dry or even quite inflamed. Many people think that such damage is an inevitable part of living and ageing, and that there is nothing you can do about it, but fortunately they are wrong. There are plenty of steps you can take to keep your skin looking healthy and beautiful.

PREPARING THE SKIN

A facial steam treatment is an excellent way of deep-cleaning the skin. Always close the pores afterwards with a skin toner, or a face mask. Keep your face about 30cm/12in above the bowl, and cover your head and the bowl with a towel for a few minutes. Steam facials should be avoided by people with thread veins.

Pore cleansers can be useful if you suffer from acne. Combine a weekly Marigold facial with a diet full of fresh, raw salad vegetables and avoid refined starches. This, combined with plenty of exercise, will relieve the skin of some of the cleansing activity (the acne) being carried out by the skin.

Steam Cleanser for Normal Skin

Put 40g/1½oz fresh or 15g/½oz dried Chamomile flowers into a bowl with 600ml/1 pint/2½ cups boiling water. Leave to stand for 30 minutes, and then strain. In a pan, re-heat the infusion and pour into a bowl. Use as directed above.

Pore Cleansers for Problem Skin

Follow the steps above, but use Marigold petals instead. Also add 5ml/1 tsp of distilled Witch Hazel to the infusion.

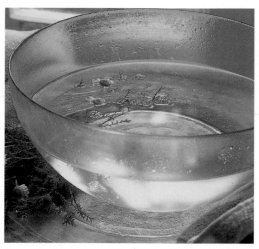

A steam treatment relaxes and softens the skin. Make it with an infusion of dried herbs, or simply float fresh herbs in boiling water.

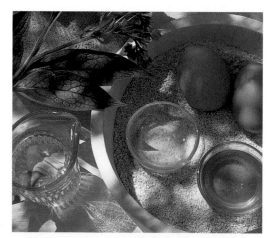

Wheatgerm oil, honey and egg yolk are all nourishing for dry skin.

FACE MASKS

Herbal face masks tighten the skin, leaving it feeling smooth and fresh. Do not use them too often as they can be over-stimulating. Comfrey and Rosewater masks are excellent for dry skin, whereas Parsley and Sage masks will help oily skin. Apply the mask mixture evenly to the face, but avoid the areas around the eyes. Leave for 10–15 minutes, and then rinse off with water.

Soothing Mask for Dry Skin

Place 6 Comfrey leaves in 150ml/¼ pint/⅔ cup boiling water, stir, cool and strain. Mix 15ml/1 tbsp of this infusion with 30ml/2 tbsp ground Wild Oats, 1 egg yolk, 5ml/1 tsp honey, 5ml/1 tsp Rosewater, 5 drops wheatgerm oil, and a little milk to mix.

Purifying Mask for Oily Skin

Infuse 15g/½oz fresh Parsley, 15g/½oz fresh Sage in 300ml/½ pint/1¼ cups boiling water. Mix 30–45ml/2–3 tbsp of this with 30ml/2 tbsp ground Wild Oats, 15ml/1 tbsp fuller's earth, 1 egg white, and 5ml/1 tsp Lemon juice.

CLEANSERS AND SCRUBS

Facial scrubs enliven the skin and encourage its self-cleansing activities. The gentle grains slough away the dead skin, stimulate the circulation and leave it looking revitalized and fresh. Scrubs are useful at any time of the year, but especially in the dark, cold winter months when skin lacks that healthy glow. They can be used in place of toner, but should be used before moisturizing the skin. Any perfumed petals, citrus skin or essential oils can be substituted into the recipes below.

To use, store the scrub in an airtight jar until it is required. When needed, mix to a soft paste with almond oil and using small circular movements, gently rub it into the skin. Rinse off with warm water and pat your face dry.

Perfumed Petal Face Scrub

Mix together 45ml/3 tbsp skinned ground almonds, 45ml/3 tbsp medium oatmeal and 45ml/3 tbsp powdered milk. Use a coffee grinder to powder 30ml/2 tbsp dried Rose petals and add them to the mixture.

Stimulating Citrus Scrub

Mix together 45ml/3 tbsp of each of the following: ground sunflower seeds, medium oatmeal, flaked sea salt and finely grated Orange peel, combine with 3 drops of grapefruit essential oil.

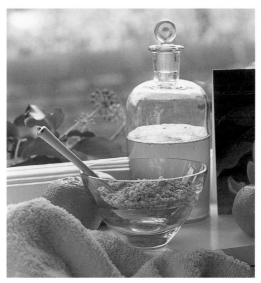

Facial scrubs are very simple to make and of all the herbal beauty treatments they keep the longest.

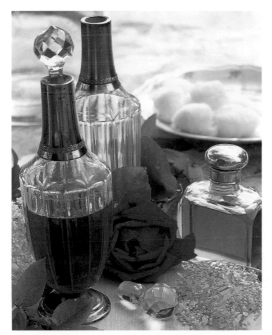

Dark red Roses are best for colour. The toner on the left is made from fragrant 'Ena Harkness', with Elderflower on the right.

SKIN TONERS

Different formulations of skin tonics are used to soothe or stimulate the skin. Fine dry skin needs soothing with delicate herbal infusions or flower waters, while large-pored or oily skins can benefit from a stimulating tonic containing witch hazel.

Orangeflower Toner for Normal Skin

Mix together 75ml/5 tbsp Orangeflower water with 25ml/1½ tbsp Rosewater. Store in a glass bottle.

Rose Petal Toner for Sensitive Skin

Place 40g/1½oz fresh Rose petals, 600ml/1 pint/2½ cups boiling water and 15ml/1 tbsp cider vinegar in a bowl. Cover and leave to stand for approximately 2 hours. Strain the toner into a clean glass bottle.

Lime Flower Toner for Mature Skin

Place 20g/¾oz fresh Lime flowers in a bowl with 90ml/6 tbsp boiling water. Leave to stand for about 2 hours then strain into a bottle. Add 10ml/2 tsp Rosewater into the bottle, shake gently and cover. This infusion will keep for 2–3 days if kept cool.

Lavender Toner for Oily Skin

Combine 20g/¾oz fresh Lavender flowers with 90ml/6 tbsp boiling water and leave to stand for about 2 hours. Strain with a sieve or through a cloth. Add 25ml/1½ tbsp Witch Hazel to the mixture, stir and decant into a bottle.

natural skin care

Your skin is the first and the most important protection you have against the outside world. If it is seen as an organ, then it is one of the body's main cleansing organs, and the one with the largest surface area. That is why it makes good sense to take excellent care of it. The simple moisturizing treatments described here will help preserve and enhance the beauty and function of your skin, keeping it in the best of health.

MOISTURIZERS

Herbal moisturizing lotions are very easy to make and require only basic kitchen tools. The herbs recommended here are a good complement to the main moisturizing ingredients, but the oils, milk, cocoa butter and beeswax are the moisturizers while the herbs add more subtle properties to the creams and lotions.

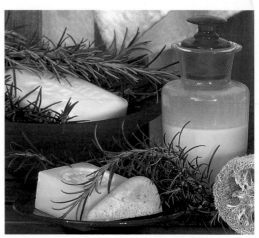

Bath Oil

Place 6 sprigs of Rosemary with vegetable oil in a jar and leave for 2 weeks, then strain. Beat together 2 eggs and 45ml/3 tbsp of Rosemary oil, then mix in 10ml/2 tbsp honey, 10ml/2 tsp baby shampoo, 15ml/1 tbsp vodka and 150fml/¼ pint/⅔ cup milk. Add 45ml/3 tbsp to the bath, and use the rest within a few days. Lemon Balm or Lavender can be substituted for the Rosemary.

Body Lotion for Dry Skin

Melt 50g/2 oz coconut oil in a heatproof bowl placed over a pan of simmering water. Stir in 60ml/4 tbsp sunflower and 10ml/2tsp wheatgerm oils. Leave to cool, then add 10 drops of Orangeflower essence and pour into a jar to solidify.

A marvellous bath lotion, made with honey and Rosemary oil, which will soon leave the skin looking healthy, smooth and silky.

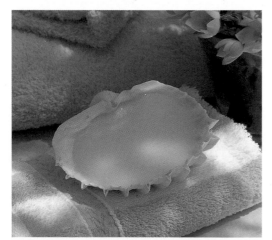

Solid moisturizers, such as this Barrier Cream, can make lovely gifts if packaged imaginatively and then wrapped in cellophane.

Instant Moisturizer

Combine 300ml/½ pint/1¼ cups almond oil with 4 drops of Rose oil, or other perfumed oil. Keep in a small bottle and use by tipping the bottle neck against the skin.

Moisturizer for Blemishes

Put 20g/¾ oz cocoa butter, 20ml/4 tsp beeswax granules and 75ml/5 tbsp almond oil in a bowl and melt over a pan of simmering water. In a separate pan, stir 10ml/2tsp borax in 175ml/6fl oz/¾ cup of Lavender water. When it has dissolved, add it to the beeswax mixture and stir to combine. Add 8 drops of Lavender essential oil, mix well and transfer to glass jars.

Barrier Cream

Grate 75g/3oz unscented soap into a bowl, pour over 90ml/6 tbsp boiling water and stir until smooth. Combine 115g/4oz beeswax, 45ml/3 tbsp glycerine, 150ml/¼ pint/⅔ cup almond oil with 45ml/3 tbsp Orangeflower water and melt in a double boiler. Remove from the heat and whisk in the soap until it thickens. Stir in 25 drops of Citrus oil and pour into containers.

HAND TREATMENTS

Gardening, winter weather, the daily grind of domestic chores and the demands of everyday living can all too easily take their toll on your hands. They can quickly become rough and sore, and even quite leathery, and the more quickly you tackle the problem the quicker your skin will become soft and supple again. This is particularly important if you like giving your partner a gentle massage. Use Roses to redress the balance.

Rose Infusion

Put a handful of fragrant Rose petals into a bowl with 600ml/ 1 pint/2½ cups boiling water. Leave for 30 minutes, pour in 30ml/2 tbsp vodka, then strain.

Rose Hand Mask

Put 45ml/3 tbsp medium or fine oatmeal, 30ml/2 tbsp Rose Infusion or triple-distilled Rosewater, 5ml/1 tsp almond oil, 5ml/ 1 tsp lemon juice and 5ml/1 tsp glycerine into a bowl and mix into a paste. Spread it on the backs of your hands and fingers and leave for 15 minutes, then rinse off with water and apply the Rose Hand Lotion.

Rose Hand Lotion

Mix together 90ml/6 tbsp glycerine, 30ml/2 tbsp Rose Infusion and 10ml/2 tsp triple-distilled Rosewater. Add 10ml/2 tsp cornflour (cornstarch) and beat until incorporated into the liquid.

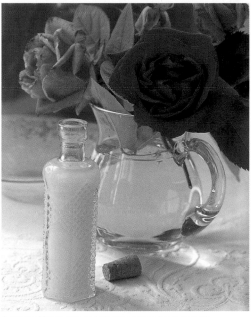

Λ lotion of Rosewater and glycerine keeps hands smooth.

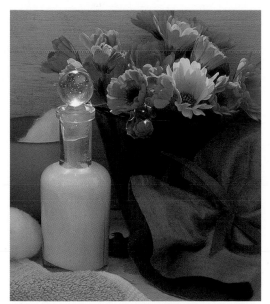

Treat inflamed skin by gently applying soothing Marigold milk to the face, dabbing it on with cotton wool balls.

TREATMENTS FOR PROBLEM SKIN

The skin can suffer from numerous complaints, from cuts and scratches to life-long eczema. Herbalism has something to offer in each case, although the latter complaint may need professional help. When using these creams, test for sensitivity by applying a little of the cream to the wrist and leaving overnight. Keep all creams in clean jars or bottles in the refrigerator.

Healing Ointment for Cuts and Scratches

Pack Marigold flowers into an airtight glass jar and leave on a sunny windowsill for 10 days. Strain off the oily liquid. Melt 90ml/6 tbsp petroleum jelly, 2.5ml/½ tsp paraffin wax and 1.5ml/¼ tsp lanolin in a double boiler. Add 10 drops of the marigold oil and mix.

Soothing Ointment for Eczema

Infuse 25g/1oz dried Comfrey, Marigold or Evening Primrose with 475ml/16fl oz/2 cups boiling water, leave for 10 minutes, then strain. In a double boiler, melt 25g/1oz beeswax with 120ml/ 4fl oz/½ cup vegetable oil, remove from the heat and whisk in 25ml/1½ tbsp of the infusion drop by drop.

Drying Tincture for Cold Sores

Place 100g/4oz dried Marigold petals with 250ml/8fl oz/1 cup vodka (30% alcohol or 60% proof). Leave for a month on a sunny windowsill. Gently shake the jar each day, then strain and store.

hair treatments

Hair is all too often taken for granted, but it too needs sensitive care and attention, particularly against the ravages of city life, with smoke and heavy pollution, and even against the worst the elements can throw at it. Store-bought shampoos can be effective, but they do lack the personal touch. You can easily achieve this by making a simple herbal treatment, which will add a wonderful attractive shine and a marvellous instant scent.

HERBAL SHAMPOOS

Much damage is caused to hair by washing it too frequently and by the detergents that it contains. This upsets the natural balance of oils and chemicals in the scalp and can create problems such as dandruff. Try these gentle shampoos instead.

Soapwort Shampoo

Break up and chop 25g/1oz fresh Soapwort root, leaves and stem or 15g/½ oz dried Soapwort root and put it into a pan. Add 750ml/1¼ pints/3 cups plain water. Simmer for 20 minutes, then strain the herbs and add a dash of Lavender water or Eau-de-Cologne. Use as ordinary shampoo.

Chamomile Shampoo

Infuse 25g/1 oz dried Chamomile flowers with 1 litre/1¾ pints/4 cups boiling water for 1 hour and then strain. Just before using mix 15ml/1 tbsp of the infusion with 60ml/4 tbsp Soapwort Shampoo and 5 drops Neroli essential oil.

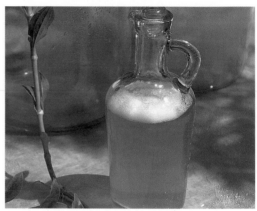

The effective cleansing properties of Soapwort (Saponaria officinalis) are due to the saponins which it contains.

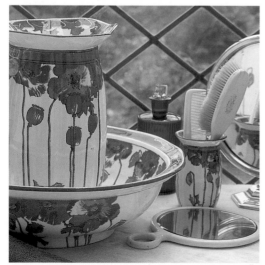

Chamomile can be used for a lightening rinse. For extra effect also add it to your shampoo.

HERBAL HAIR RINSES

For keeping the hair shiny and to enhance its natural colour, try using the following rinses after shampooing. Simply stand over a bowl and pour through the hair and re-apply at least 6 times.

Chamomile Rinse for Fair Hair

Infuse 25g/1oz dried Chamomile in 1 litre/1¾ pints/4 cups boiling water. in a large bowl for 1 hour, and then strain.

Rosemary Rinse for Dark Hair

Infuse 40g/1½ oz fresh Rosemary in 1 litre/1¾ pints/4 cups boiling water in a bowl for 1 hour and then strain.

Nettle Rinse for Dandruff

Infuse 25g/1oz fresh Nettle leaves in 1 litre/1¾ pints/4 cups boiling water overnight then strain. Add 30ml/2 tbsp cider vinegar and 30ml/2 tbsp Witch Hazel.

Herbal Remedies	
• Chamomile	• Rosemary

caring for the mouth
Commercial mouth treatments are often harsh and contain chemicals that can affect the self-balancing and self-healing abilities of the mouth. Toothpastes may also contain detergents which can adversely affect the lining of the gut, and this can also cause problems. If you have time it is worth making your own tooth powders and mouthwashes, which can be adapted, when needed, to treat any upsets in the mouth.

ORAL HYGIENE
The mouth is often one of the first places that tells us when we are run down. The most common symptom of this is mouth ulcers, and oral thrush is also quite common. The first priority to aid prevention and recovery is to eat plenty of fresh vegetables, raw and cooked, and have enough exercise and plenty of rest. Secondly, use a simple tooth powder or paste that will not interfere with the natural balance of good bacteria in the mouth that help to fight simple infections.

Tooth Powder
Bake 25g/1oz fresh shredded Sage or Mint leaves with 60ml/4 tbsp sea salt or orris root at a very low temperature in the oven for 1 hour. Pound the mixture to a fine powder and use on a damp toothbrush. Note that if you are pregnant or planning a pregnancy, Sage should be avoided.

Tooth Cleaners
Simpler herbal tooth cleaners include fresh Sage leaves rubbed over the teeth or Lemon peel can be rubbed over teeth to remove stains.

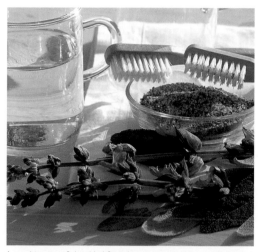

A combination of shredded Sage leaves mixed with sea salt, baked and then powered, is traditionally used for cleaning teeth.

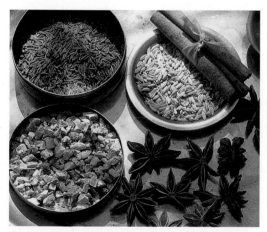

Chewing various seeds and spices to freshen and sweeten the breath is a widespread custom in the Far East.

BREATH FRESHENERS
Bad breath or halitosis is often symptomatic of a digestive problem or the onset of a cold and therefore may require the help of a professional herbalist or doctor. At other times, it is simply the result of eating too much garlic or spicy food. Whichever it is, this recipe will sweeten your breath.

Refreshing Mouthwash
Simmer 5ml/1 tsp each of ground nutmeg, ground cloves, cardamom pods, caraway seeds and 15g/½oz dried Lemon Balm with 600ml/1 pint/2½ cups purified water. Strain and add 30ml/2 tbsp sweet sherry. Store in a clean bottle. Dilute 15–30ml/1–2 tbsp in a glass of water.

Breath Enhancers
The following fresh herbs and dried spices can be chewed to freshen breath: Parsley, Watercress, Mint, seeds of Fennel, Star Anise, Cinnamon stick or cloves. Alternatively rinse your mouth with diluted rosewater.

guide to herbs and their uses It has long been

known that herbs are an essential part of the kitchen, adding all kinds of flavours, and for helping to relieve and cure a range of problems from migraines to wind (gas). The early physic gardens in monasteries were really basic pharmacies stocking many of these essential plants. Do not try and compete. Just grow those herbs that you know will help you feel much better.

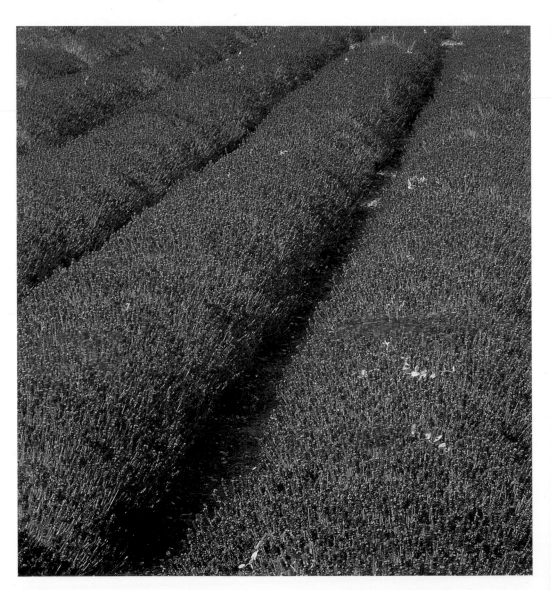

USING HERBS

The herbs described on the following pages are a particularly useful group for helping tackle stress and various other common conditions. Reading the notes and studying the pictures will help you decide which would be most beneficial for you and your garden. After all, they should also help make a special relaxing feature. If planting them in groups, remember to put the tallest in the centre and the smaller ones around.

You may well want to try several as remedies before deciding which you find most helpful. Note that herbs do not usually work instantly, so do not be impatient and give them at least two weeks to take effect. If you do not feel better in three weeks, seek the help of a qualified practitioner. Herbs can also be used in various combinations, and you will find suggestions for putting them together to give additional benefits.

Since most of us would benefit from a nerve tonic during stressful times, choose the herbal remedy best suited to you.

For example, if when stressed you start to feel depressed, then look for a stimulating herbal tonic such as Wild Oats. If, however, stress makes you feel anxious and you start developing symptoms such as palpitations, sweating and sleeplessness, then turn to those herbs that have a relaxing effect.

Rescue Remedy, because it is not strictly herbal, but a Bach Flower remedy is not included in this directory, but it is readily available over the counter.

It is quite clear that some herbs are multi-talented. Borage gives a marvellous show of flowers and adds to the cottage garden, attracting plenty of bees. The leaves add a cucumber flavour to drinks, the flowers can garnish salads, and the oil lowers blood pressure. Lavender is another all-purpose herb, essential for pot-pourris and for a range of soothing treatments. If you find some plants do not succeed in certain parts of the garden, move them around until you find a more suitables place and you may well find that they perk up.

LADY'S MANTLE
Alchemilla xanthochlora syn.
A. vulgaris, Virgin's Cape

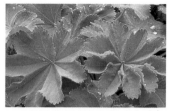

The unusual leaves of this plant resemble a cloak, hence its common names. The name Alchemilla derives from the Arabic word for alchemy, signifying its power to help make a change. A larger species, Alchemilla mollis, is grown as a foliage plant. Lady's Mantle is a women's herb and helps balance menstrual cycles. As a douche or wash, an infusion helps sooth any itching or inflammation.

n o t e s • Parts used: Leaves and flowers.
• Dose: I tsp dried/2 tsp fresh to a cup of boiling water three times a day.

PASQUE FLOWER
Anemone pulsatilla, Wind Flower

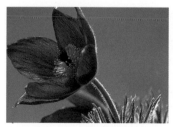

One of the most beautiful medicinal herbs with purple spring flowers. The common name comes from *Pasch* meaning Easter. Pasque Flower is a sedative, bactericidal, anti-spasmodic painkiller used to treat the reproductive organs. It is used against all types of pain affecting male and female genital organs.

n o t e s • Parts used: Dried leaves and flowers.
• Dose: A very low dose is needed – it is advisable to consult a herbalist.
c a u t i o n : Do not use the fresh plant.

MUGWORT
Artemisia vulgaris

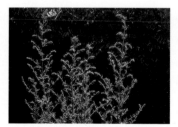

The "mother of herbs" grows robustly along roadsides and is said to protect the traveller. It is best described as a tonic with particular application to the digestive and nervous systems; it reduces nervous indigestion, nausea and irritability. As a womb tonic it helps regulate the menstrual cycle, reduces any associated period pain and PMS. It is also used to repel insects, including moths.

n o t e s • Parts used: Flowers and leaves.
• Dose: ¼–½ tsp three times a day.
c a u t i o n : Avoid in pregnancy.

WILD OATS
Avena sativa

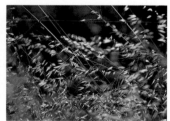

Oats are an excellent tonic to the nervous system. They slightly stimulate and are a long-term remedy for nervous exhaustion. They also help cope with shingles and herpes. Oats contain vitamin E, iron, zinc, manganese and protein and help reduce cholesterol.

n o t e s • Parts used: Seeds and stalks.
• Dose: There are many ways to take oats – in gruel, porridge, flapjacks, oatcakes and other dishes, as well as tea.
c a u t i o n : Oats are not always suitable for those who are sensitive to gluten.

BORAGE
Borago officinalis

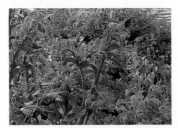

A strapping plant with lovely, luminous blue flowers. They make an attractive garnish to ice cream and cold summer puddings. Borage boosts the production of adrenaline and is useful in times of stress. It is also very nutritious, and helps to treat skin diseases and rheumatism.

n o t e s • Parts used: The leaves, flowers and seeds. The leaves need to be dried quite quickly and are best heated very gently in a cool oven until they are crisp.
• Dose: 1 tsp dried/2 tsp fresh to one cup of boiling water.

CHAMOMILE
Chamomilla recutita or
Chamaemelum nobile

This pretty daisy is one of the better known herbs, possibly because it is so useful. Use the flowerheads alone in a tea or tincture to relax both the digestive function and those gut feelings that may sometimes disturb you. It makes a very suitable tea to drink late in the day because it has quite the opposite effect to that of coffee, which actually exacerbates tension and anxiety.

n o t e s • Parts used: Flower heads.
• Dose: 1 tsp dried/2 tsp fresh to a cup of boiling water.

CALIFORNIAN POPPY
Eschscholzia californica

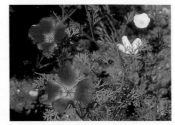

The beautiful, delicate flowers last for one day and are then replaced by long pointed seed pods. The stunning hot orange, yellow and pinkish colours of the blooms might account for its French name, *globe de soleil*. Californian Poppy is a gentle painkiller and sedative which reduces spasms and over-excitability.

n o t e s • Parts used: The whole plant
• Dose: 1 tsp dried herb to a cup of boiling water.
c a u t i o n : It is important to avoid this herb if you suffer from glaucoma.

LICORICE
Glycyrrhiza glabra

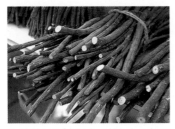

A highly useful herb which has been cultivated since the Middle Ages for its sweet, aromatic roots. It aids digestion and reduces inflammation along the gut, loosening the bowels. Licorice heated in honey makes a soothing syrup, helping to soothe attacks of bronchitis and asthma.

n o t e s • Parts used: The root (Licorice sticks) or solidified juice in the form of black bars.
• Dose: 1 tsp to a cup of boiling water.
c a u t i o n : Not recommended for those with high blood pressure or oedema.

HOP
Humulus lupulus

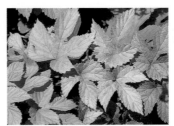

The name Hop comes from the Anglo-Saxon *hoppen*, "to climb": the twining fibrous stems may top 4.5m/15ft. Hops are taken as a bitter tonic helping both to improve digestion and to reduce any restlessness. It also has a sedative effect and will provoke deep sleep. The action is partly due to its volatile oils.

n o t e s • Parts used: Dried flowers from the female plant, called "strobiles".
• Dose: Not more than 1 tsp a day.
c a u t i o n : Avoid the use of Hops during any depressive illness.

ST JOHN'S WORT
Hypericum perforatum

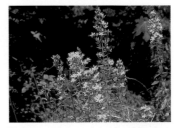

To be sure that you have the right plant, hold a leaf to the sun; the oil glands look like little holes. The plant is now well known for its anti-depressant action. It is a nerve tonic which helps nervous exhaustion and damage to nerves caused by diseases such as shingles.

n o t e s • Parts used: Flowering tops.
• Dose: 1 tsp dried/2 tsp fresh to a cup of boiling water, three times a day.
c a u t i o n : This remedy is best avoided when you are spending any time out in the garden when there is bright sunlight.

GINSENG
Korean Ginseng, *Panax spp.*

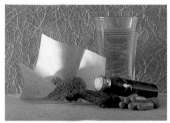

By improving the production of adrenal hormones, Korean Ginseng helps the body to adapt to stress and resist disease. It should only be taken for short periods though. It benefits ME sufferers.

n o t e s • Parts used: Dried root.
• Dose: 1g per day.
c a u t i o n : Avoid the use of Ginseng during pregnancy or when taking other stimulants. Do not take high doses for more than six weeks without seeking expert advice. Stop taking Ginseng if it makes you feel agitated or if you develop a headache.

LAVENDER
Lavandula spp.

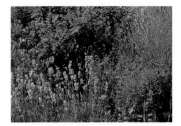

Everybody knows this fragrant plant. Herbalists call it a thymoleptic, which means it raises the spirits. This, combined with its anti-infective action and relaxing properties, makes Lavender a powerful remedy. The essential oil is used externally for relaxation and to heal sores and burns. Lavender can also be taken internally in a tea or tincture. It is also an ideal remedy for irritation, indigestion and for the onset of a migraine attack.

n o t e s • Parts used: Dried root.
• Dose: 1g per day.

MOTHERWORT
Leonurus cardiaca

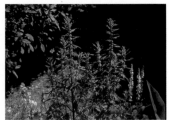

The Latin name refers to the leaves shaped like a lion's tail. It is a great calmer if tension is causing palpitations or sweats. It improves the circulatory system and is also used to relieve any menstrual and menopausal problems. Motherwort can also help to lower blood pressure.

n o t e s • Parts used: Leaves and flowers.
• Dose: 1 tsp dried/2 tsp fresh to a cup of boiling water three times a day, or 2 tsp syrup.
c a u t i o n : It is important that it is avoided in the first trimester of pregnancy.

LEMON BALM
Melissa officinalis, Bee Balm

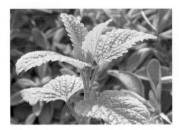

This plant has so much vitality that it can spread all over the garden. It makes a suitable drink for every day; hot in winter and iced in summer. Lemon Balm aids digestion and relaxation, and sensitive digestive systems. It is much used for irritable bowels, nervous indigestion, anxiety and depression. It makes a good bedtime drink, promoting peaceful sleep and a sense of relaxation.

n o t e s • Parts used: Leaves and flowers.
• Dose: 1 tsp to a cup of boiling water, taken up to three or four times a day.

MINT
Mentha spp.

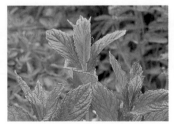

Peppermint (Mentha piperita) is a hybrid between Spearmint and Watermint. It is antiseptic and anti-parasitic, and will reduce itching. It has a temporary anaesthetic effect on the skin and gives the impression of cooling. It is included in lotions for massaging aching muscles, and makes an effective footbath.

n o t e s • Parts used: Leaves and flowers.
• Dose: 1 tsp dried/2 tsp fresh to a cup of boiling water.
c a u t i o n : It is important that it is avoided in the first trimester of pregnancy.

EVENING PRIMROSE
Oenothera biennis

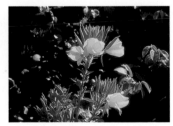

A beautiful plant, luminous in the twilight, which freely self-seeds in the garden. It is used externally for eczema and other dry skin conditions. Taken internally, Evening Primrose oil reduces cholesterol levels and benefits the circulation. It has a decent success rate on women with PMS, and can help calm hyperactive children. It also helps regenerate livers which have been damaged by alcohol.

n o t e s • Parts used: Oil from seeds.
• Dose: Capsules as directed.
c a u t i o n : Avoid in cases of epilepsy.

MARJORAM
Origanum vulgare

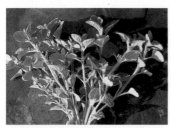

There are many species of Marjoram, and they are used in potpourris and cooking. Medicinally, Marjoram reduces depression and helps tackle nervous headaches. It contains volatile oils which are antispasmodic, making it useful when soothing digestive upsets. The infused oil can be used in the bath to relieve stiffness, or rubbed on to soothe sore and aching joints or muscles.

n o t e s • Parts used: Leaves.
• Dose: I tsp dried/2 tsp fresh to a cup of boiling water, taken twice a day.

PASSION FLOWER
Passiflora incarnata, Maypop

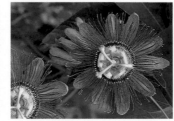

This is a climbing plant which produces spectacular flowers. It is often included in sleeping mixes, and is very helpful when tackling restlessness and insomnia. It counteracts the effects of adrenaline, which may cause anxiety, palpitations or nervous tremors. It is used to ease the pain of neuralgia.

n o t e s • Parts used: Dried leaves and flowers.
• Dose: ¼-½ tsp dried herb twice a day, or I tsp at night, or take an over-the-counter preparation as directed.

ROSEMARY
Rosmarinus officinalis

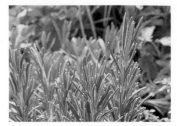

A familiar plant containing several active, aromatic oils. Like Lavender, it can be used both externally, in the form of an essential or infused oil, and internally as a flavouring, tea or tincture. The actions of Rosemary are centred on the head and womb. It increases the supply of blood to both. In the head it helps tackle cold headaches and in the gut eases spasms due to poor circulation.

n o t e s • Parts used: Leaves and flowers.
• Dose: I tsp to a cup of boiling water taken up to three times a day.

SAGE
Salvia officinalis

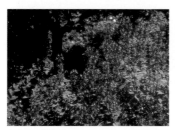

A beautiful, evergreen plant with fine purple flowers in early summer. Like many culinary herbs, it aids digestion. It has antiseptic properties and can be used as a compress on wounds that are slow to heal, or as a gargle or for infections of the mouth or throat. It is also said that it will help reduce night sweats and menopausal hot flushes, and can darken greyish hair.

n o t e s • Parts used: Leaves.
• Dose: I tsp dried per cup of boiling water.
c a u t i o n : Avoid during pregnancy.

SKULLCAP
Scutellaria lateriflora

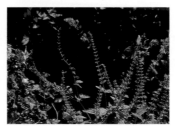

This herb is another nervous tonic. It was traditionally associated with the head, because it produces skull-like seed pods. It is very calming. Skullcap can help reduce anxiety and restlessness. Its bitter taste encourages the liver to remove toxins from the body, as well as excess hormones which can cause degrees of premenstrual tension.

n o t e s • Parts used: Aerial parts, which are harvested after flowering.
• Dose: I tsp dried/2 tsp fresh to a cup of boiling water.

WOOD BETONY
Stachys betonica syn. S. officinalis, Betonica officinalis, Bishop's Weed

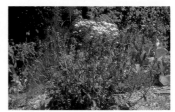

An attractive plant with purple flowers. Wood Betony aids the nervous system, especially if sick headaches and poor memory are a problem. It also encourages blood flow to the head. Always a popular remedy throughout Europe, it is certainly well worth trying if you get headaches or migraines.

n o t e s • Parts used: Aerial parts.
• Dose: I tsp dried/2 tsp fresh herb to a cup of boiling water.
c a u t i o n : It is important that you avoid high doses during pregnancy.

LIME BLOSSOM
Tilia × europaea, Linden Blossom

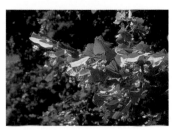

The tall upstanding Lime tree has honey-scented blossom. Medicinally it is relaxing and cleansing. It makes a helpful tea for fevers and flu, especially if combined with Yarrow and Peppermint. It encourages sweating and aids the body through fevers. It is also used to reduce hardening of the arteries and high blood pressure, and to relieve migraines.

notes • Parts used: Flowers, including the pale yellowish bracts.
• Dose: I tsp dried/2 tsp fresh to a cup of boiling water taken three times a day.

DAMIANA
Turnera diffusa

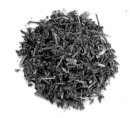

Damiana grows in South America and the West Indies. It was previously called Turnera aphrodisiaca and is a tonic to the nervous and reproductive systems. It is useful if the sexual function is impaired. It is taken as a remedy by men, but the stimulant and tonic work equally well for women. Damiana is harvested when in flower, and is dried for use as an anti-depressant, and to relieve anxiety.

notes • Parts used: Leaves and stem.
• Dose: 2 tsp to a cup of boiling water, which can be taken twice a day.

VALERIAN
Valeriana officinalis, All Heal

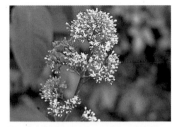

This is a tall herb with whitish-pink flowers which grows in damp places. The root has a powerful sedative effect on the nervous system, and effectively reduces tension. It can be used to reduce period pains, spasms, palpitations, and hyperactivity. It is good if anxiety makes sleep difficult.

notes • Parts used: Dried root.
• Dose: I tsp to a cup of boiling water at bedtime.
caution: High doses taken over a long period may cause headaches.

VERVAIN
Verbena officinalis, Herb of Grace

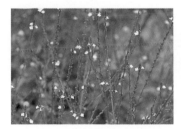

An unassuming plant with tiny flowers. Vervain is a nervous tonic with a slightly sedative action. It is useful for treating nervous exhaustion and symptoms of tension which include headaches, nausea and migraine. It has a bitter taste and has been used for gall bladder problems. It is quite often recommended for anyone who has depression, and works well with Wild Oats.

notes • Parts used: Leaves and flowers.
• Dose: I tsp dried/2 tsp fresh to a cup of boiling water.

CRAMP BARK
Viburnum opulus, Guelder Rose

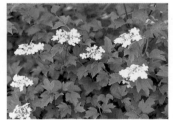

A decorative wild bush which produces glorious white and pale pink spring flowers, followed by autumn red berries. Writer Geoffrey Grigson said it had a smell like crisply fried, well-peppered trout. Therapeutically, the use of Cramp Bark is a good illustration of the connection between body and mind. It reduces spasms whatever the cause and helps tackle constipation, period pains, and high blood pressure.

notes • Parts used: Dried bark.
• Dose: I tsp to a cup of boiling water.

CHASTE TREE
Vitex agnus-castus, Monk's Pepper

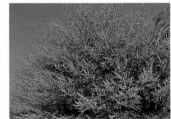

The common name reflects a slight anti-oestrogen effect which can cool passion: perhaps this property may account for its other common name, Monk's Pepper. Small doses of this herb can re-balance the hormones and reduce some of the symptoms of PMS, menopausal change, infertility, post-natal depression and irregular periods. It also increases milk production after birth.

notes • Parts used: Dried ripe fruits.
• Dose: 10–20 drops of tincture which are taken first thing in the morning.

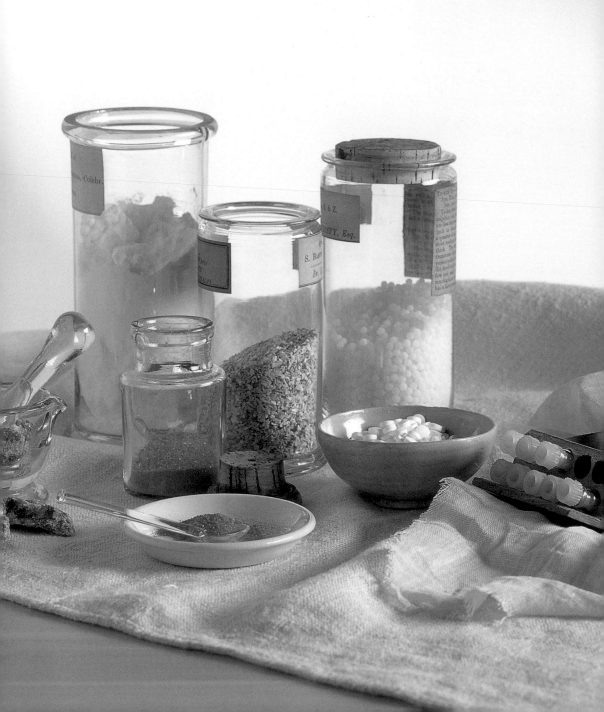

homeopathy
homeopathy

homeopathy

The name "homeopathy" was coined by Samuel Hahnemann from two Greek words meaning "similar suffering", or "like cures like". Appalled by the savage medical practices of the day, Hahnemann, a German doctor and chemist, started on a course of study that led to the development of homeopathy. His philosophy of disease and its cure through natural processes has changed very little from that day to this. The traditional approach is today's approach.

The principle of like curing like, or "the law of similars", as it is sometimes called, decrees that if a substance can cause harm to a healthy person in large doses, it also has the potential to cure the same problem in tiny doses by stimulating the body's own natural energy, enabling it to heal itself.

The law is best illustrated by example. In the 19th century it was a custom among German women to take the herb Valerian as a stimulant. The practice was abused and overtaxed the nervous system. Yet, given in minute doses, Valerian relaxes the nervous system, and is one of homeopathy's main remedies for insomnia.

The doses used in homeopathy are so minute that they cannot be acting directly on the physical body. Hahnemann considered that what they did was act dynamically: in other words, the energy of the remedy stimulated the natural healing energy of the body. If it had been in a state of disharmony, then it would be propelled back to its former, healthy state.

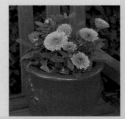

homeopathy and health

Homeopathy is not only an energy medicine, it is also holistic. Homeopaths convincingly argue that the body is much more than the sum of its various parts, and that the mind, the emotions and indeed the organs are somehow intricately interconnected. Consequently, the treatments they give are more "rounded" than those found in traditional medicine. They are not just aimed at the symptom, but at the whole person.

ENERGY WITHIN

The mechanics of this interconnection are elaborate and hard to explain, but it is clear that the process really does work. The key point is that underlying the physical and mental systems of the body is a refined system of energy which is self-regulating. It generally works extremely well. You sense it in action when you become ill. We usually get better even without taking a medicine. The body heals itself though it might need support when its own natural energy is low.

Treatment

The healing process is like running a car. Modern cars are so efficient that, provided you maintain them properly, give them the right fuel and drive them sensibly, problems seldom arise. Then one night you forget to turn off the lights and the next morning the battery is flat and your car incapacitated. The only way to get it moving again – the only cure – is to get a transfer of energy, in the form of a jump start from another battery. Homeopathy is in many ways just like getting an energizing jump start.

Homeopathy is becoming increasingly popular because of the serious concerns about drugs-based orthodox medicine. Many drugs are toxic and the side-effects in susceptible people can actually be quite unpleasant. Even if the side-effects are not observable, the long-term consequences from the excessive use of drugs are not always fully appreciated. In fact modern medicine seldom cures, and it does not even pretend to. What it does do is alleviate and palliate the symptoms, and manage the illness, but since it addresses the symptoms and rarely the cause, the results are not entirely satisfactory.

Homeopathy is different because it is safe and it does not treat the removal of symptoms as an end in itself. Symptoms are considered as signs of distress or adjustment. The correct remedy removes the cause of the problem; the symptoms will then fade away. Homeopathy is highly rated because it takes into account the nature of the person. It knows that when two people have been diagnosed as having the same illness, they can actually become ill in quite different ways and will require different remedies to effect a satisfactory cure.

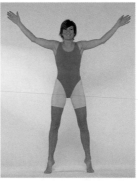

Sometimes our bodies just do not seem to be firing on all cylinders, and we need a carefully chosen homeopathic boost to revive them.

DEFINING DISEASE

We become ill when our energy is depleted or when we are out of harmony. In fact the word "disease" could be more accurately written "dis-ease", indicating that we are definitely not at ease, and for a disease to be cured it is not necessary to give it a name. To cure homeopathically depends on a sensitive, accurate analysis of the symptoms. There is usually no need for a diagnosis, for it is widely said that there are no diseases, only what might be called people who are "dis-eased".

Symptoms

Except for any life-threatening situations, symptoms are not the primary problem. They reflect a picture which shows how the system is making adjustments to heal itself. For example, both diarrhoea and vomiting are the body's way of ridding itself of unwanted "material", and the intolerable itching of eczema does not specifically mean that you have a skin disease. Rather it means that there is an imbalance in your whole system, and that your body is pushing the problem to the safest possible place, well away from the essential organs. The skin becomes an organ of elimination.

Treating the Whole Person

Some people are very robust and seldom become ill, others are over-sensitive and become run-down and sick after a slight chill or an emotional upset. For some, the chest is the greatest weakness: winter colds quickly turn to bronchitis. With others digestion is the problem: the slightest unusual change to their diet causes an immediate upset. Homeopathy acknowledges these many differences and adjusts all treatments accordingly. The professional homeopath will always prescribe "constitutionally" to try to strengthen the weak areas, as well as the whole system.

Causes of Illness

There are many causes of disease. Some are obvious, such as being run-down and poor nutrition, but illness might have an emotional cause. Stress creates disharmony which manifests itself in physical ailments. Homeopathy takes such factors into account and, if possible, tries to mitigate them and strengthen the sufferer.

Reading the Symptoms

When trying to cure a disease, the vital force causes the body to produce symptoms. Homeopaths call this "the symptom picture". These symptoms accurately reflect exactly what is happening inside, and they also indicate what outside help or extra energy is therefore now required.

For example, during a flu epidemic two children in the same family become ill. The first child catches the flu very suddenly, overnight, and develops a high fever with a red face and a dry burning heat all over the body. The second child's symptoms might be very different, appearing quite slowly over several days. This child's fever is much lower, but he is shaky and shivery and his muscles ache all over. Both children have the same flu, but the vital force has produced completely different symptoms. Each child therefore needs to be treated in quite a different way. The homeopath will certainly understand this and give the first child the remedy Belladonna, while the second child receives quantities of Gelsemium. Homeopathy is well known for excelling at individualizing such treatments.

While it is quite true to say that in homeopathy we do not treat symptoms but the individual sufferer, we are still extremely interested in the symptoms. For it is through careful observation of the complete symptom picture that we can discover which remedy is required. In acute ailments the vital force will eventually effect a cure, given sufficient time, but by giving a helping hand from an accurate reading of the symptoms, that is by giving the body an "energy fix", the process can in fact be speeded up considerably.

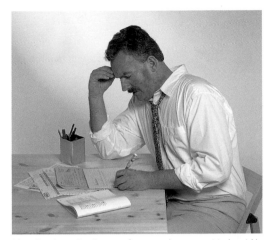

Mental and emotional stress, often at work, can surprisingly quickly lead to a range of physical problems.

CHRONIC DISEASES

With so much battering from within and without, it may seem a wonder that we are not all permanently ill. Of course, many people are. Although many of the acute infectious diseases of the past have ceased to be a serious problem, their places have now been taken by today's chronic diseases. Never has there been so much cancer and heart disease, eczema and asthma, or even digestive problems such as irritable bowels. Our immune systems are overstretched in combating these problems.

The Immune System

It is all too easy to ignore the incredible adaptability and intelligence of the immune system, which appears to make heroic efforts to keep us up and running despite considerable adversity. One writer shrewdly called this intelligence the "vital force". He described it as "the spirit-like force which rules in supreme sovereignty". It has also been well described as "the invisible driver", overseeing the checks and balances that are needed to keep us in the best possible health.

The Vital Force at Work

Most of the time we are completely and utterly unaware of this sophisticated balancing process which is entirely automatic and pre-programmed through our genetic make-up. We can certainly observe it in action when we contract an acute illness (i.e. one that arises suddenly) such as a fever or a cough. What we may not always realize is that the fever is really a necessary, natural function and that it actually "burns up" the infection, and that the cough exists to prevent any active accumulation of mucus in the lungs. The body is extremely resourceful. However, chronic diseases (i.e. those that develop slowly, or are of long duration) might well need outside help, and a consultation with an experienced, professional practitioner.

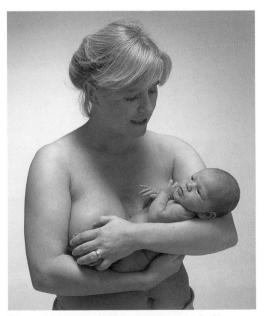

We are all born with a vital force that oversees our health.

using remedies

When first taking a homeopathic remedy, you might well be totally bewildered how anyone could possibly know that a certain recipe of mixed ingredients is the one that is best for you. In fact there is no guesswork. The exact remedies for all kinds of problems have been known and listed for hundreds of years. The technique is precise and proven, and the beauty of it is that remedies can be subtly fine-tuned to suit your particular ailment.

REMEDY SOURCES

The remedies used in homeopathy are derived from many sources. The majority are prepared from plants, but many minerals are also used and a few remedies are even prepared from insect and snake poisons and other toxic substances. Do not be alarmed about the toxins because they have been diluted so that no danger remains. The Law of Similars shows that the most powerful poisons can be turned into equally strong remedies. In fact about 2,000 have now been described and documented, but in practice most professional homeopaths use only a fraction of that surprisingly high number.

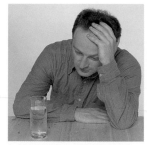

In homeopathy every symptom is fully taken into account when trying to apply the right remedy.

The process that turns a substance into a remedy is called "potentization", and consists of two main procedures, dilution and succussion (or vigorous shaking). When you buy a remedy note a number after its name, usually 6, but also other numbers rising in a scale: 30, 200, 1M (1,000). Sometimes a "c", standing for centesimal (one hundredth) appears after the number. It shows how often the remedy has been diluted and succussed.

A remedy is prepared by dissolving a tincture of the original material, usually in alcohol. On the centesimal scale, the 6th potency means that the original substance has been diluted six times, each time using a dilution of one part in a hundred. This results in a remedy that contains only one part in a million million of the source material. Yet the greater the potency (number of dilutions), the greater the remedy's power.

Between each dilution, the remedy is succussed. When the potentization is complete the remedy is preserved in alcohol, and a few drops can be added to a bottle of milk-sugar pills or a cream. The remedy is now ready to use.

PROVINGS

Almost all homeopathic remedies have been "proved", or tested, although practitioners gain additional knowledge of them from clinical experience. In a proving, a remedy is tested on a group of healthy people over a period of time, until they develop symptoms. Neither the supervisor nor the group should know what remedy they are proving. This is a double blind test, conducted on sound, regulated principles. The symptoms that the provers develop are accurately collated until a complete symptom picture has been obtained. Consequently, we know exactly what the remedy can cure.

Once proved, remedies can be used for all time. Hundreds of original remedies are still in use today. The remedy pictures are described in great detail in volumes called *Materia Medica*. Because thousands of symptoms for thousands of remedies have been proved over the last 200 years or so, no one homeopath could possibly remember them all. They are therefore listed in another impressively detailed book called *The Homeopathic Repertory*. It is, in effect, an index to the *Materia Medica*. Between them, these two astonishing books cover most symptoms.

In homeopathy, physical examinations are seldom necessary, but bright, sparkling eyes are a sign of good health.

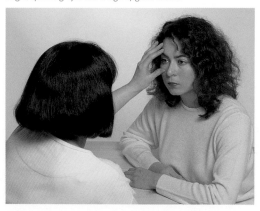

Tissue Salts

The 19th-century German doctor Wilhelm Schussler identified 12 vital minerals, or "tissue salts", essential to health. According to his theory, many diseases are associated with a deficiency of one or more of these substances, but they can be cured by taking the tissue salts in minute doses, singly or in all kinds of different combinations.

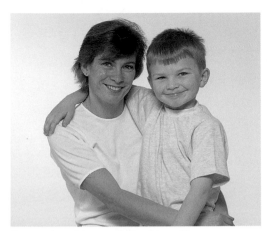

Even members of the same family will have different susceptibilities to illness and react differently

CHOOSING THE CORRECT REMEDY

With a copy of the *Materia Medica*, the homeopath is now well equipped to match the symptoms with the symptom picture. This is usually known as finding the similimum (or similar).

The Symptom Picture

Finding the correct remedy is like trying to arrange a perfect marriage. If the two partners are compatible, success is almost certain. If the remedy is a good match to the symptoms, the patient is going to feel a good deal better, the natural way. The words "I feel better in myself" are like music to the ears of the prescribing homeopath, because it means that the natural healing processes have been stimulated successfully, even if some of the physical symptoms remain. It should be only a short time before they too disappear.

The prescriber is like a detective looking for clues. Apart from the obvious general symptoms, such as fever, headache or a cough, you should note what are called the "modalities" – that is, what aggravates or alleviates the symptoms, or makes the person feel generally better or worse. They might include the need for warmth, or cool air, sitting up or lying down. Notice whether the person is thirsty or sweaty; whether the tongue is coated, and the state of the breath. What kind of pain is it: throbbing, stitching or sudden stabs of intense agony?

It is also important to note if the symptoms have an obvious cause? Did they arise after an emotional shock, or after catching a chill in a cold wind? Did they arise dramatically and suddenly in the middle of the night, or have they developed in rather a nondescript way over a number of days?

It is also very important to note the person's state of mind. For example, irritable people who just want to be left alone may need quite different remedies from those who want to be comforted and are easily consoled. The homeopath has to be sensitive in all kinds of ways.

HOW TO USE REMEDIES

Many minor and self-limiting acute problems can be treated safely at home with a basic first-aid kit. However, for more serious long-term ailments, or if you feel out of your depth and really worried – especially if young children or old people are ill – seek help from your own homeopath or doctor. Access to professional homeopaths is now much easier, and they can often do wonderful things for persistent and chronic disease. Be assured that qualified practitioners will have completed three or four years' training.

What the given remedy is doing is helping your body to help itself. Sometimes there may not be a great deal you can do – a well-established cold is going to mean several days of suffering whether you intervene or not. In other cases, the sooner you act, the better: for instance, if you take Arnica (either in pill form, or rubbed-in cream if appropriate) immediately after a bad fall for the bruising and shock, the results will be very impressive with the healing time being be much shorter.

You can often limit the duration or intensity of suffering, as in fever, sepsis (pus-forming bacteria), pain, indigestion and many other conditions. Moreover, there will be many satisfying times when the problem is aborted or cured altogether.

Once you are confident of an improvement then the vital force needs no further help, and you can stop taking the remedy. You will do no harm if you do in fact carry on, but there is really no point in trying to acquire far more energy than your mind and body actually require. In homeopathy it is perfectly true to say that less is actually more.

You may feel rather hesitant and uncertain about treating very young children, but it is known that homeopathy usually works extremely well on them, and can be safely used from birth.

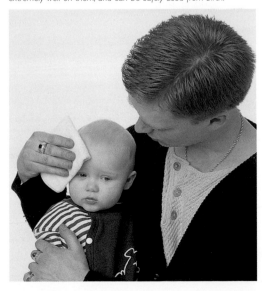

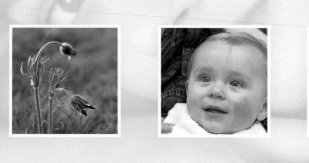
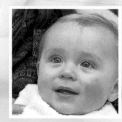
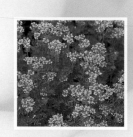
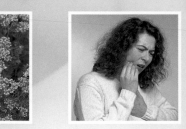

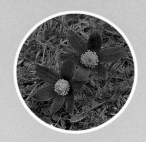

remedies for common ailments
remedies for common ailments

remedies for common ailments

Many straightforward problems can be treated at home using homeopathy. For each one, the following pages list a number of remedies that are likely to be the most helpful in the situation. Read the remedy picture carefully and choose the one that best seems to match the symptoms that you have observed. Then, when you have selected your own particular remedy, double-check it very carefully with the more detailed description which you will find listed in the Materia Medica section. Rescue Remedy is often used by homeopaths, though it is not strictly homeopathic, for that reason it has not been included in the Materia Medica.

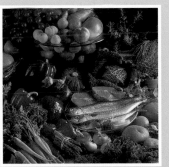

How to Take the Remedy

Carefully empty one pill into the cap of the bottle. If more than one tumbles into the cap, tip the others back into the bottle without touching them. This is quite important. If you are shaky, use a folded piece of paper to help if necessary.

Next, drop the pill on to a clean tongue – that is, you should take the remedy at least ten minutes before or after eating, drinking or cleaning your teeth. The pill should be sucked for about thirty seconds before being crunched and swallowed. Remedies for babies can be crushed to a powder in an envelope and given on a teaspoon.

Giving the Remedy

The 6th and 30th potencies are most useful for home use. As a rough rule of thumb, use a 6c three or four times a day, or a 30c once or twice daily until symptoms improve. One pill at a time is all that is necessary; there is no need to reduce the dosage for children.

In serious situations such as a high fever or after an accident, you can give a remedy every half-hour if necessary. Since the active content of the remedy is so small, you cannot overdose in acute situations and if you do not get a good reaction within a day or overnight, you may want to consider a second remedy. Never worry about giving the wrong remedy: it will either work or it will not. If it does not work you will have done no harm to the patient.

Sometimes the symptoms may change after giving a remedy, so that a new picture emerges. You then need to find a new remedy to fit the new picture. If the situation improves, or the picture is unclear, watch and wait. Only intervene if you feel you need to.

Until you get used to the method of diagnosis, you may find it helpful to consult a practitioner on the first few occasions, this is also a good idea if symptoms persist. The Homeopath will also be able to give other effective advice.

colds, flu and toothache

Most colds, unless nipped in the bud, take their natural course and they should clear up in about week. Even so, they can make life pretty uncomfortable, as can a throbbing toothache. Flu, however, can be much more debilitating, though a good remedy can often help ameliorate the symptoms, soon reducing the effects of aching bones, weak legs, headaches, high temperatures, shivering and even dizziness.

Colds and Flu

If flu comes on suddenly, often at night and perhaps after catching a chill, with symptoms of high fever and profuse sweating, Aconite is a perfectly good remedy. If the symptoms are similarly sudden and with a high temperature, but accompanied by redness, burning heat and a headache, then the remedy is much more likely to be Belladonna.

For flu that appears more slowly, accompanied by extreme thirst, irritability and the desire to be left alone, Bryonia will be very useful. Probably the most widely used remedy in flu, though, is Gelsemium. The most pronounced symptoms are shivering, aching muscles and general weakness. Where aching bones are prominent, use Eupatorium.

For head colds with sneezing and an acrid nasal discharge, Allium cepa or Arsenicum should be very helpful. If the sinuses are also affected and there is a lot of yellow-green mucus which appears in globules, or if it looks sticky and stringy, then use quantities of Kali bich.

For a general tonic, both during and after the flu, when your symptoms are not very well defined and there is a general feeling of malaise, try using Ferrum phos.

Kali bich can be a good remedy for blocked sinuses where there is pain and a green stringy discharge.

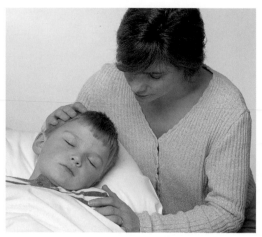

The most useful remedies at the start of a high fever in children are Aconite and Belladonna.

Fevers

Fevers, particularly in children, whose temperatures may be quite high, may seem alarming, but it should be remembered that they are the body's own efficient, natural response to dealing with and burning up infection.

The two main remedies for high fevers that appear suddenly are Aconite and Belladonna. Thirst and sweat characterize the Aconite picture, while Belladonna cases will reveal a dry skin, redness, and a throbbing pain in the affected area. If the fever appears more slowly and the person is irritable, wants to be left alone and is very thirsty for cold water, try Bryonia. For flu-like fevers, with shivering, weakness and aching muscles, use Gelsemium. Ferrum phos can be used in milder fevers, with no particularly distinctive symptoms. Pulsatilla is really useful in children's fevers, where the child soon becomes very emotional, clingy and weepy, and wants to be comforted.

If the period of fever is made more uncomfortable by poor circulation and chilblains, the former can be helped by herbs that stimulate the circulatory system. Angelica and Ginger have a good track record, taken with the likes of Yarrow. The latter is best treated by a tincture of Arnica.

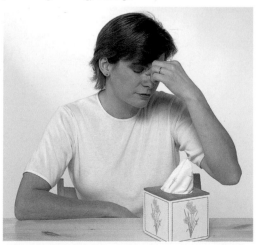

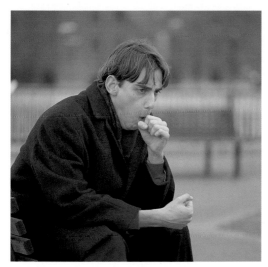

At the first sign of a head cold, try Arsenicum or Allium cepa.

Coughs and Croup

For very harsh, dry, violent coughs, which may appear suddenly and may be worse at night, use Aconite. For a hard, dry painful cough, which seems to be helped by holding the chest very tightly and also by long drinks of cold water, use Bryonia.

For deep-seated, dry, spasmodic coughs that may end in retching or even vomiting, use Drosera. Painful, barking coughs, which produce thick yellow-green mucus, may be helped by Hepar sulph. For coughs that are really quite suffocating, and which sound sharp and rasping, like a saw going through wood, try Spongia. Where there is a lot of mucus seemingly trapped in the chest, try Ant tart.

Croup is a horrible sounding dry cough that affects small children. The main remedies are Aconite, Hepar sulph and Spongia. Try each one of these remedies in turn if it is in any way difficult to differentiate between the symptoms.

Sore Throats

If a sore throat starts suddenly, often during the night, perhaps following a chill and accompanied by a high temperature, try Aconite. If the throat burns and throbs painfully and looks very red, it may be eased by Belladonna.

For a sore throat that looks very swollen and puffy, with a stinging pain, try Apis. Hepar sulph can be used for an extremely painful throat that feels as if there is a fish bone stuck in it, making it very difficult to try and swallow.

If the sore throat feels worse on the left side and swallowing liquids is particularly painful, use Lachesis. Use Lycopodium if the throat is worse on the right side or the pain moves from right to left; warm drinks may be comforting.

For a sore throat which is accompanied by offensive breath and saliva, with a degree of sweatiness and thirst, then you should try Mercurius. For throats that appear dark, raw and red, and feel as if a highly uncomfortable, unpleasant hot lump has got stuck inside, try taking quantities of Phytolacca. That usually proves quite effective.

Relieving Toothache

There is probably no worse agony than the pain of toothache, as the area is so sensitive. In most cases, a visit to the dentist will be essential, but the following remedies may well help you cope with the pain in the meantime.

For sudden and violent pains, perhaps precipitated by a cold, Aconite may be helpful. If the area looks very red and throbs violently, Belladonna should be used. For abscesses, where pus is obviously present and the saliva tastes and smells foul, the best remedy is likely to be Mercurius. If you are prone to abscesses and your teeth are generally not very strong, Silica should be used to strengthen the system.

For pain that lingers after a visit to the dentist, take Arnica or Hypericum. If the pain is in any way accompanied by extreme irritability, Chamomilla should be used.

Hepar sulph is a suitable remedy for extreme septic states (infected areas), where bad temper is a prominent symptom. Another remedy for toothache where there are spasmodic shooting pains is Mag phos.

Though there are several remedies that can help with toothache, you will still need to visit the dentist.

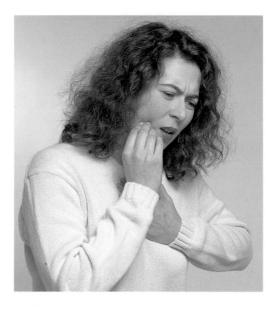

eyes and ears
Any problems with the eyes and ears can be immediately quite distressing, especially for young children who do not appreciate what is happening. Their world can suddenly be turned upside down. Fortunately, there is a wide range of proven remedies for helping ease such discomfort, for example reducing puffy, swollen eyes, styes, burning sensations, and even the debilitating effects of a sudden, throbbing ear infection.

SOOTHING THE EYES

Overwork, pollutants, viral and bacterial infections can all affect the delicate tissues in and around the eyes. Stress and fatigue tend to aggravate these problems by weakening the immune system's ability to fight off infection.

Aconite helps when the eye feels hot and dry, perhaps after catching a cold. The eye may feel irritated, as if it has got a piece of grit. Apis is a good remedy to use when the eyelids look puffy and swollen; the discomfort can be reduced and relieved by applying a cold compress.

Belladonna is a very good remedy for eyes that look in any way red and bloodshot, and which are over-sensitive to light. Euphrasia is one of the very best remedies for sore and burning eyes, and it can also be used in an eyebath because it can be obtained in a diluted tincture.

One of the best remedies for styes is Pulsatilla, which should be used when the eye has an infection which results in what is best described as a sticky yellow discharge. When treating eye injuries, Symphytum can be used where there has been a blow to the eyeball. For general eye injuries, Arnica will ease the bruising. Ledum helps when the eye is cold and puffy.

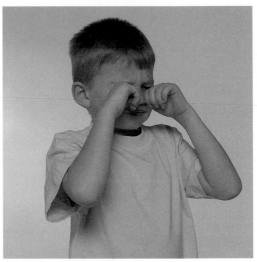
Eye irritants cause a lot of discomfort and need tackling quickly.

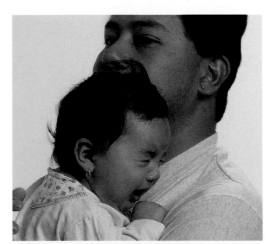
An effective cure for children's earaches is Verbascum oil.

EAR INFECTIONS

Acute earaches are most common in young children. They need to be treated quickly, as an infection within the middle ear can be both painful and damaging. Speedy home help can be very useful, but you must get professional medical help if the earache worsens or if it in any way persists.

One of the most soothing remedies is Verbascum oil. Pour a few drops into a spoon that has been pleasantly warmed, and drip gently into the child's ear.

For sudden and violent pains, accompanied by fever which usually start at night, use Aconite. Where there is a fever with a sudden and violent appearance, and the ear throbs and looks very red, Belladonna will effect a cure.

For earaches where there is great pain and the child is exceptionally irritable, use Chamomilla. Ferrum phos is required where the pain comes on slowly and there are no other significant distinguishing symptoms. For very painful, sore earaches with some discharge of yellow-green mucus, when the child is also clearly chilly and irritable, use Hepar sulph.

allergies

Over the last 20 or 30 years there has been a highly significant increase in all kinds of allergies, which might be better described as the body's sensitivity to an excess of substances that cannot be easily assimilated. Sadly, many such substances are the product of our time. Hay fever, eczema, asthma, irritable bowel disease and other chronic diseases have now reached almost epidemic proportions. Fortunately, homeopathy can offer you essential help.

HAY FEVER

Hay fever is rather a misnomer, for there are many other substances apart from hay which can trigger the well-known symptoms of watering eyes and runny nose, itchiness and sneezing. The problem may last for a few weeks, a few months or even all year, depending on the cause.

Euphrasia and Allium cepa are two of the most effective acute remedies. If the problem is centred in the eyes, with even the tears burning, Euphrasia is the remedy to use. However, if the nasal symptoms are worse, with constant streaming and an acrid discharge, then try Allium cepa. Another remedy that is sometimes useful when there are constant burning secretions from the mucous membranes is Arsenicum.

To build up your immune system, it is best to act about two to three months before the time when hay fever usually begins. There are plenty of tasty aids. Garlic, in pill form or meals when it can even be eaten whole if roasted in the oven, imparting a new, sweetish flavour, works well. So too do regular applications of honey. Inhaling over a steam bath using lemon balm reduces the chances of an allergic attack.

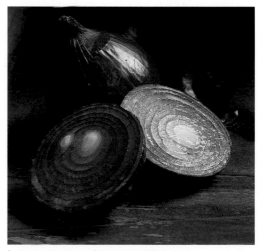

Red onion, the source of the remedy, Allium cepa.

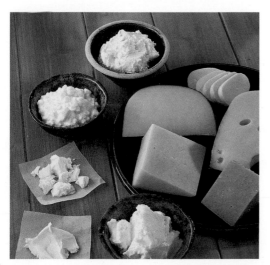

CHRONIC DISEASES

No one knows precisely what causes these problems. Further research is required. Quite clearly there are many different reasons. Toxicity overload is almost certainly one. The body simply cannot cope with the increasingly large number of chemicals and drugs that it was never designed to absorb. Another likely reason is deficient nutrition. Many of our foods are now so over-processed (apart from being sprayed with all kinds of chemicals) that they do not contain sufficient minerals and vitamins to allow the body to function efficiently.

Homeopathy can often work wonders in correcting the many weaknesses that result from such causes. Obviously, you should also take care to avoid toxic substances wherever possible, and eat a healthy, varied diet. The homeopathy that is needed to cure chronic ailments is complex and beyond the scope of this book; seek advice from a professional homeopath.

Allergies, or over-sensitivity to certain foods, are becoming increasingly common. Research shows that dairy products and wheat-based foods seem to cause the most problems.

acute illnesses and upsets

There is nothing quite as frustratingly disabling as a sudden upset stomach, whether it be diarrhoea, lingering indigestion, niggling cramps or even quite painful bouts of trapped wind. But with the use of homeopathy you do not have to keep on suffering. It actually offers several well-proven ways of helping you tackle such problems, so that you can resume a normal life, quickly getting out and about.

SETTLING GASTRIC UPSETS

The main symptoms of stomach and intestinal infections are pain, wind (gas), nausea, vomiting and diarrhoea. Bear in mind that vomiting and diarrhoea are actually natural processes by which the body rids itself quickly of any unwanted material. Consequently these symptoms need to be treated only if they are persistent. Such problems can arise at any time and may be due to food poisoning or just a sudden reaction to unfamiliar food; this invariably seems to happen on vacation.

Upset Stomach

The great standby remedy is Arsenicum. Other symptoms which may accompany diarrhoea or vomiting are excessive weakness, coldness and restlessness. Mag phos is an excellent remedy for general abdominal cramps which are soothed by doubling up and making sure that you keep warm.

For constant nausea which is unrelieved by vomiting, use Ipecac. Nux vomica is a very good remedy for gastric upsets where nothing really seems to happen. The undigested food lies like a horrible dead weight in the stomach and refuses to move or be expelled, causing plenty of discomfort.

Phosphorus can be a useful remedy for diarrhoea, and it is particularly effective if attacks are accompanied by a sensation of burning in the stomach. While you may crave a cold drink, it is actually vomited as soon as it warms up in the stomach.

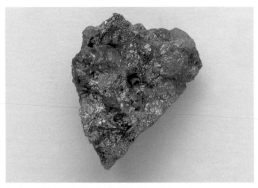

A piece of Arsenopyrite used in the remedy Arsenicum.

Indigestion

The symptoms of indigestion are heartburn, wind (gas) and cramping pains. They are usually caused by eating too much or in fact eating too quickly. The symptoms are usually much more marked when you are eating very rich food and drinking large quantities of alcohol. The most useful remedy is Nux vomica. The digestive system seems heavy and sluggish and the feeling is that you would be much better if the undigested food would move. Another good remedy that can help is Lycopodium.

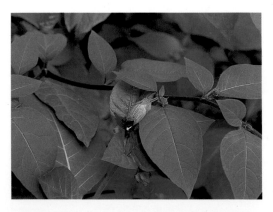

CALMING BOILS AND ABSCESSES

Sometimes, an area of skin becomes inflamed and gathers pus. This usually happens around a hair follicle. The build-up of pus can cause acute pain before it comes to a head as a boil or abscess, or until the pus is absorbed by the body.

In the early stages of a boil or abscess, when it looks red and angry and throbs painfully, Belladonna is often the best remedy. Later when it starts becoming septic (infected) and even more painful as the pus increases, use Hepar sulph. If the boil seems very slow in coming to a head, Silica should be used to speed up the process. This remedy is also helpful as a daily tissue salt for unhealthy skin that keeps producing boils. The nails may also be unhealthy, breaking and peeling too easily.

Belladonna is highly effective against a wide range of complaints.

emotional issues
We underrate at surprisingly great risk the incredible part that our emotions can play in our health. Diseases can easily arise from any disharmony in our lives. This is even more likely if we are repressed, unable to express and articulate our more difficult, upsetting emotions, feelings staying trapped and locked within us. Just as joy can bolster and keep us in good health, a big build-up of grief can result in all kinds of illness.

Emotional Turmoil
It is not unusual for a homeopathic practitioner to hear words like "I've never really got over my father's death," or "I've never properly felt well since my divorce." It is important for good health not to allow such wounds to fester. Homeopathy can often help chronic and acute conditions when needed.

In any emotional situation where you feel that you really cannot cope, the Bach Flower Rescue Remedy is useful. Although it is not strictly homeopathic, it works well with homeopathic remedies, and can be taken as often as you wish.

Grief and Fright
Ignatia is the number-one remedy for acute feelings of sadness and loss. It can calm both the hysterical and over-sensitive and those who tend to keep their grief bottled up. Children and emotionally dependent people can be helped by Pulsatilla. Aconite is considered the major remedy for helping people who need to get over a shock or a terrifying experience.

Anticipation
The worry brought on by a forthcoming event such as an exam, appearing on the stage or meeting someone new can severely affect some people. Fortunately, there are a number of remedies that can help ease any anxiety and panic.

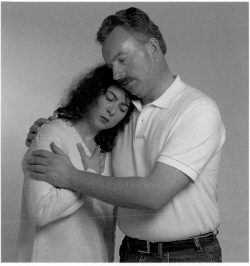

The most useful remedy for dealing with emotional upsets is Pulsatilla, combined with plenty of security and love.

Gelsemium is best used when you start trembling with nerves and literally go weak at the knees. Arg nit is a good all-round anxiety remedy, where there are symptoms of great restlessness. It also has a claustrophobic picture and could help those who suffer from a fear of flying or even travelling on underground trains. The panic often causes diarrhoea, and another anxiety remedy that can help the bowels is called Lycopodium. Strangely, people who need Lycopodium are often found to excel at the ordeals that they have been worrying about, once they have overcome the panic barrier.

Insomnia
There can be many causes of sleeplessness including worry, habit, and bad eating. For the "hamster on the wheel" syndrome, where your mind is rushing around in never-ending circles, Valerian can be a magical aid helping you quickly fall asleep. For those sufferers who constantly wake too early, especially if they are people who live too much on their nerves and eat large quantities of rich food, try Nux vomica.

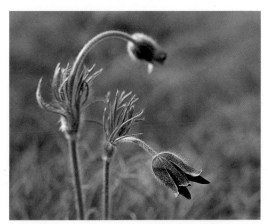

A Pasque flower, used in Pulsatilla.

women's health
Two of the greatest concerns to most women are their reproductive systems and the effects of their associated hormones, but many find they are treated in quite a heavy-handed way by traditional modern medicine. Fortunately, homeopathy offers another route and a range of different treatments which can include important aspects of your diet. Homeopathic self-help can ease the distress for various non-persistent conditions.

Anaemia
Anaemia is usually caused by an iron deficiency and manifests itself through weakness, pallor and lack of stamina. The most vulnerable times are during pregnancy or after excessive blood loss due to heavy periods. Since iron pills supplied by your doctor can often severely upset the bowels, gentler methods are actually preferable. Eat foods rich in iron and try organic iron preparations which can be obtained from health food shops. Ferrum phos should also be used on a daily basis.

Cystitis
Many women are familiar with the burning agony of urinating when they have a bladder infection. Cranberry juice or sodium bicarbonate can often help. Two of the most useful remedies are Cantharis and Apis. Use Cantharis as a general remedy. Apis can be helpful when the last drops in urination hurt the most.

Mastitis
Mastitis means an inflammation of the breast and it occurs commonly during breast-feeding. It can be painful but is not normally serious. Fortunately, breast-feeding does not have to stop because of it. Homeopathy is usually very successful in curing the inflammation. Phytolacca is the most important remedy aiding breasts that may feel lumpy and swollen.

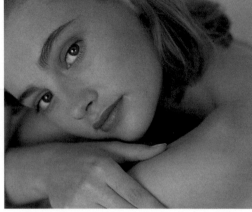

PMT mood swings are not uncommon and should not alarm you. Check your symptoms to find a remedy that might help.

Pre-menstrual Syndrome (PMS)
Most women are familiar with the mood changes that arise just before an oncoming period. For an unfortunate few, more extreme symptoms of depression, anger and weepiness can appear, sometimes as much as a week or more before the flow begins. A visit to a professional homeopath can certainly be of great benefit, but there are several remedies that you might like to try yourself at home in order to alleviate some of these sudden, extreme symptoms.

Pulsatilla is an excellent remedy if weeping and the feeling of neediness is prominent. Sepia should be used where there is anger and exhaustion, and even in cases of indifference towards your family. Lachesis is very helpful in minimizing the more extreme symptoms of violent anger, jealousy and suspicion.

Period Pains
If your period pains are consistently bad, you will need to consult a homeopath. For occasional pains, there are a number of self-help remedies from which you can choose. The three PMS remedies mentioned above, Pulsatilla, Sepia and Lachesis, should be considered when applicable, and if your symptoms seem significant and over-riding. All three might also be of some help during a difficult menopause.

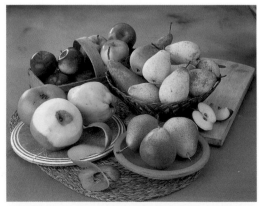

A good diet is essential for good health. Fresh organic apples and other fruit are especially good for you.

children's health

Children tend to respond very well and quickly to all kinds of homeopathic treatments, and they are a joy to treat. However, while there is actually no substitute for constitutional treatment from a professional homeopath who will try to boost the immune system as much as possible, there is no reason why you should not keep a good stock of remedies at home in case of a sudden, acute situation. You too can do a lot to help.

Children and Homeopathy

The best start you can possibly give a child is plenty of confidence, with love and security, breast milk for as long as is practical, a healthy, varied diet, as few drugs as possible, and homeopathy. Young children invariably have rather dramatic, acute conditions, such as fevers. Usually there is nothing for you to worry about if you are well informed, have professional support and have access to remedies. The dosage is the same as for adults, but remember to crush the pills first for babies.

Teething

The most widely used remedies for teething pains are Chamomilla and Pulsatilla. Chamomilla is an "angry" remedy and suits bad-tempered babies best. These are the ones that drain you of sympathy because you have had so many sleepless nights making you feel irritable and guilty for becoming bad tempered, and helpless. Only constant attention, picking them up and carrying them round, soothes them in any way. Pulsatilla children respond differently – they are softer, weepy and are constantly in need of your sympathy. They feel better and are significantly soothed by being given plenty of cuddles.

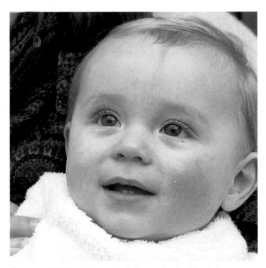
Give your child the right start with love and a healthy diet.

For babies, it is essential to crush the tablet first.

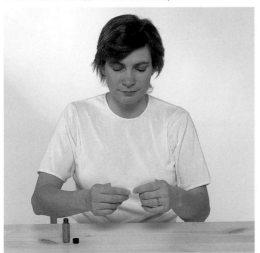

Fevers

Many small children get fevers with very high temperatures, as they burn up infection in the most efficient way. Seek help if the fever goes on for more than 24 hours, especially if there are any signs at all of a violent headache or drowsiness. Aconite and Belladonna are the best, general high-fever remedies.

Croup

This harsh, dry cough is very disturbing in small children, but usually sounds far worse than it really is. There are three main remedies for croup. Aconite can be used for particularly violent and sudden coughs, which are often worse at night. For harsh coughs that sound like sawing through wood, Spongia is the remedy. For a rattly chest with thick yellow-green mucus, possibly marked by irritability and chilliness, use Hepar sulph.

Colic

Trapped wind can be very upsetting for a baby. It comes without warning, and for no apparent reason the baby will cry. Sometimes babies try to curl up to ease the pain, and warmth and a gentle massage should help. Mag phos is a useful remedy to try.

first aid

Homeopathic remedies are extremely useful as first-aid treatments in all kinds of situations, but dangerous, serious injuries should always receive immediate, expert medical attention. If you are in any way alarmed or concerned, you must first call for help, at which point it might just be possible to start giving an appropriate remedy. In more minor cases, such as bruising, cuts and sprains, homeopathy can certainly make quite a difference.

Bruises

The very first remedy to think of after any injury or accident is Arnica. For local bruising, where the skin is unbroken, apply Arnica cream, and whether you use the cream or not you can give an Arnica pill as often as you think necessary, until such time as the bruising starts to go down.

Arnica is also wonderful in cases of shock. If the person is dozy or woozy, or in fact unconscious, crush the remedy first and place the powder directly on to the lips.

Where there is serious shock, or in any real emergency, use Rescue Remedy. This can be used either alone or with Arnica in cases of physical trauma. Place a few drops of the Rescue Remedy straight on to the lips or tongue, every few minutes if considered necessary. If the injury results in pains shooting up the arms or legs, try using Hypericum.

This remedy is also very useful where sensitive areas have been injured and hurt, such as the toes, fingers, lips and ears. If the joints or bones have been hurt, Ruta may be more effective than Arnica, which is more of a soft tissue remedy.

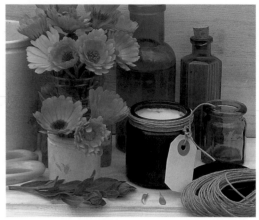

Calendula cream is a widely available, excellent remedy to use if you have got any open cuts and sores.

Cuts, Sores and Open Wounds

Clean the area thoroughly to remove all dirt. If the wound is deep, it may need stitches and you must seek instant medical help. Once the wound is clean, apply some Calendula cream.

Puncture Wounds

Such injuries can easily occur in all kinds of ways: from animal or insect bites, pins, needles and nails, and even from standing on a sharp instrument such as a garden fork or rake.

If the wound becomes puffy and purple and feels cold, with the pain being eased by a cold compress, Ledum is the best remedy. If there are shooting pains, which travel up the limbs along the tracks of the nerves, then Hypericum should be used.

Sprains, Strains and Fractures

For general muscle strains, resulting from lifting heavy weights or excessive physical exercise such as aerobics or long hikes over hilly countryside, Arnica will almost always be extremely effective. For deeper injuries where the joints are affected, as a result of a heavy fall or a strong football tackle, use Ruta.

For even more severe sprains, especially to the ankles or wrists, where the pain is agony on first moving the joint but eases with gentle limbering up, Rhus tox should be very helpful. For injuries where the slightest movement is extremely painful and hard pressure eases the pain, Bryonia will provide relief.

Once a broken bone has been set, use Symphytum daily, night and morning, for at least three weeks. This will not only ease the pain but speed up the healing of the bones.

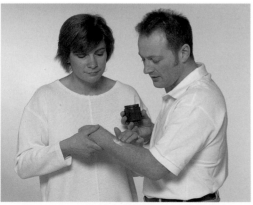

For bites that come up as any kind of bruise, small or dramatic, apply Arnica cream. For many it is very effective.

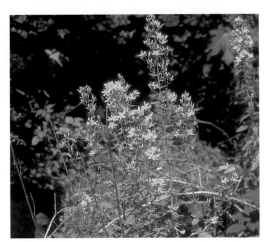

The herb St John's Wort, used in the remedy Hypericum.

Burns

Severe burns need urgent medical assistance: do not delay, especially in the case of children and babies. For minor burns and scalds, Calendula or Hypercal cream can be very soothing, especially if applied straight away. If the pain remains, or the burn is severe, take one pill of the remedy Cantharis every few hours until the pain eases. In the case of shock or a hysterical child, also use Arnica (in pill form) and/or Rescue Remedy.

Bites and Stings

For minor injuries, you can apply Calendula or Hypercal cream. If the wound looks in any way bruised, use Arnica, either as a cream or in pill form. However, if the wound becomes dramatically swollen and starts looking red and puffy, then use Apis. For any injuries to quite sensitive areas, such as the fingers, especially when shooting pains can be felt, Hypericum is a useful remedy. Ledum is preferable if the wound looks puffy and feels cold to the touch, and is helped by the application of a cold compress.

Travel Sickness

Many people end up getting seasick even when the waves are not too rough, and some, especially children, are also air-sick or car-sick. The symptoms are eased by the remedy Cocculus.

Fear of Flying

Use Aconite and/or Rescue Remedy before you go to the airport and then as often as you need during the flight. If you actually find yourself shaking with anxiety, try Gelsemium. If the problem is more a question of claustrophobia, the fear of being trapped in a narrow space, Arg nit should be very useful.

Visits to the Doctor or Dentist

For any pre-visit nerves, to which we are all prone at some time, take Arg nit. For surgery or dental work where bruising and shock to the system might well have been involved, you cannot go wrong with Arnica. Take one pill before the treatment, and one pill three times a day for as long as you actively need it.

The Homeopathic First-aid Kit

It is a good idea to keep a basic first-aid kit in the house so that you are well prepared for any sudden emergency. Many remedies are now available from health food shops and even some chemists, but for many of us there might not be a nearby source, and it is amazing how many emergencies arise outside shop-opening hours. Stock up and be safe.

Your first-aid kit should include:
Arnica cream – for bruises
Calendula cream – for cuts and sores
Echinacea tincture – for the immune system
Rescue Remedy tincture – for major emergencies

Although not strictly a homeopathic treatment, Rescue Remedy is one of Dr Edward Bach's Flower Remedies. These flower essences are a series of gentle plant remedies which are intended to treat various emotional states, regardless of the physical disorder.

Plus these bottles of pills:
Aconite – for fevers, coughs and colds
Apis – for bites and stings
Arnica – for bruising or shock following accidents
Arsenicum – for digestive upsets and food poisoning
Belladonna – for high fever and headaches
Bryonia – for dry coughs and fevers
Chamomilla – for teething and colic
Ferrum phos – for colds, flu and anaemia
Gelsemium – for flu and anxiety
Hepar sulph – for sore throats and infected wounds
Hypericum – for injuries

Ignatia – for grief and emotional upsets
Ledum – for puncture wounds, bites and stings
Lycopodium – for anxiety and digestive problems
Mercurius – for sepsis
Nux vomica – for hangovers, nausea and indigestion
Phosphorus – for digestive problems and nosebleeds
Pulsatilla – for ear infections, fevers and eye problems
Rhus tox – for sprains, strains and rashes
Ruta – for injuries to tendons and bones

the materia medica

There are something like 2,000 remedies in the homeopathic Materia Medica, though most of them are actually best left to the professional practitioner. However, there are a surprising number of remedies that can safely be used by the lay person in low potencies for acute and first-aid cases. These remedies cover a wide range of not too serious, non-persistent problems. It is well worth seeing just how much you can achieve.

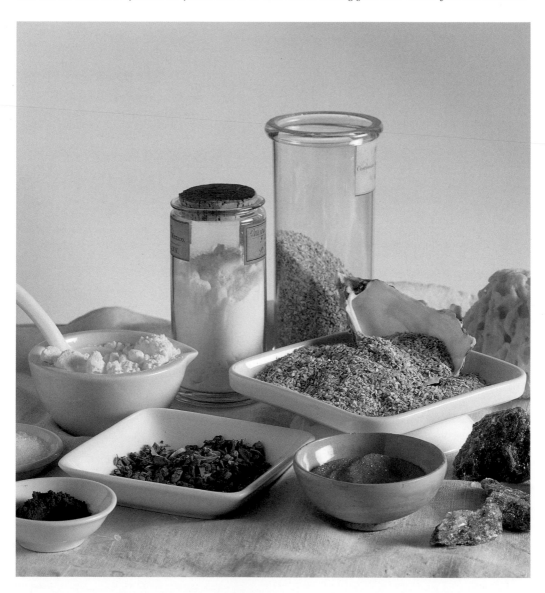

HOMEOPATHIC CURES

Use this section to back up and confirm your choice from the remedies that were recommended for ailments earlier in the chapter on herbs. If your choice still looks good, then you are almost certainly on the right track. However, if it does not, then consider trying one of the other remedies which are described for the ailment. Do note, though, that not every particular symptom of the remedy has to be present. Homeopaths use the expression "a three-legged stool"; if the remedy covers three symptoms of the condition, then it is more than likely to be well indicated.

Note that you must always keep your supply of remedies in a cool, dark place or cupboard. Also do keep them well away from any strong, pervasive smells and young children. Fortunately, homeopathic remedies are known to be extremely safe, so even if a child does actually swallow a number of pills, even as much as a whole bottle, you need not be unduly alarmed or concerned.

ACONITE
Aconitum napellus

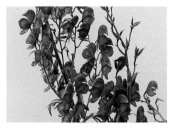

Monkshood, a beautiful yet poisonous plant with blue flowers, is native to mountainous areas of Europe and Asia. It is widely cultivated as a garden plant.

n o t e s • Symptoms appear suddenly and violently, often at night. • They may appear after catching a chill or after a fright. • Fear or extreme anxiety may accompany symptoms. • An important remedy for high fevers with extreme thirst and sweat. • Major remedy for violent, dry croupy coughs. • It is most effective when used at the beginning of an illness.

ALLIUM CEPA
Allium cepa

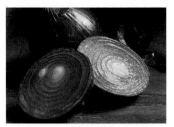

The remedy comes from the onion, whose characteristics are perfectly well known and obvious to anyone who has ever had to peel a strong one: it directly affects the mucous membranes of the nose, the eyes and throat.

n o t e s • Sneezing, often repeatedly, accompanied by a streaming nose. • The nose and eyes begin to burn and become irritated. • Nasal discharge is acrid while the tears are bland. • Major remedy for hay fever (when the nose is affected more than the eyes) and also for colds.

ANT TART
Antimonium tartaricum

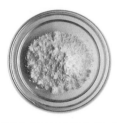

Ant tart is prepared from the chemical substance antimony potassium tartrate, and is traditionally referred to as tartar emetic. Ant tart affects the mucous membranes of the lungs.

n o t e s • A wet, rattling cough from deep in the lungs, with shortness of breath and wheezing. • Helps to bring up mucus from the lungs.

APIS
Apis mellifica

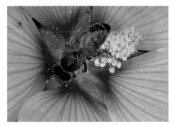

The remedy is prepared from the honey bee. The well-known effects of its sting describe the remedy picture very well.

n o t e s • A useful remedy after injuries, especially from bites or stings where there is subsequent swelling, puffiness and redness. • The affected area feels like a water bag. • A fever appears quickly and without any thirst. • The person appears restless and irritable. • The symptoms are often relieved by the application of a cold compress, or exposure to cold air.

ARG NIT
Argentum nitricum

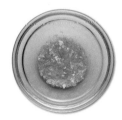

Silver nitrate, from which this remedy is derived, is one of the silver compounds that are used during the photographic process. It is good at helping to soothe an agitated nervous system.

n o t e s • Panic, nervousness and anxiety. • Feeling worried, hurried and without emotional and practical support. • Fears of anticipation which might include stage fright, exams, visiting the dentist, flying, and many others. • The nervousness may cause diarrhoea and wind (gas).

ARNICA
Arnica montana

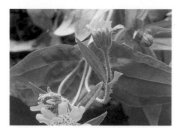

Arnica is a well-known herb with yellow, daisy-like flowers. Its native habitat is mountainous areas. It has a special affinity with soft tissue and muscles, and is usually the first remedy to consider after any accident. Where there is bruising but the skin is not broken, use Arnica cream. (When the skin is broken, use Calendula or Hypercal cream.)

n o t e s • The most important remedy for bruising. • Shock following an accident. • Muscle strains after strenuous or extreme exertion.

ARSENICUM
Arsenicum album

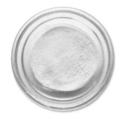

Arsenic oxide is a well-known poison. However, when used as a homeopathic remedy it is extremely safe and works especially well on the gastro-intestinal and respiratory systems.

n o t e s • Vomiting, diarrhoea, abdominal and stomach cramps. • Often the first remedy in cases of food poisoning. • Asthmatic, wheezy breathing, often worse at night. Head colds with a runny nose. • Chilliness, restlessness, anxiety and weakness. • Warmth gives great relief.

BELLADONNA
Atropa belladonna

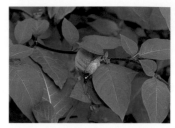

The valuable remedy Belladonna must be prepared from deadly nightshade, whose poisonous berries are best avoided. However, they produce a medicine which is one of the most important fever and headache remedies.

n o t e s • Violent and intense symptoms appearing suddenly. • Fever with high temperature, little thirst and burning, dry skin. • The face or the affected part is usually bright red. •Throbbing pains, especially in the head. •The pupils may be sensitive to light.

BRYONIA
Bryonia alba

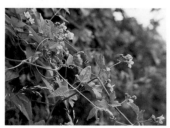

Bryonia is prepared from the roots of white bryony, a climbing plant which is found in hedgerows right across Europe. The roots are surprisingly large and store a great deal of water. Bryonia patients often seem to lack "lubrication".

n o t e s • The symptoms tend to develop slowly. • Dryness marks all symptoms: in the mouth, membranes and joints. • Extreme thirst. • The condition feels worse with the slightest motion.• Bryonia coughs are dry and very painful. • The person is irritable.

CALENDULA
Calendula officinalis

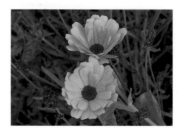

Calendula has long been known to herbalists as a major first-aid remedy for injuries. It is prepared from the common marigold, and the simplest way to use it is as a cream. When combined with Hypericum it is known as Hypercal.

n o t e s • Use this cream on all cuts, sores and open wounds. (For bruises where the skin is not broken, use Arnica cream.) • Calendula is a natural antiseptic and keeps the injury free of infection, as well as helping to speed up the healing process.

IPECAC
Cephaelis ipecacuanha

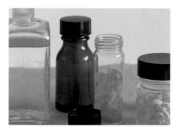

Ipecacuanha is a seemingly small, insignificant South American shrub. The remedy works mainly on the digestive and respiratory tracts, and the most important symptom it treats is nausea, no matter what the ailment.

n o t e s • Persistent nausea, not helped by vomiting. • Coughs that are accompanied by feelings of nausea. • Outbreaks of morning sickness during pregnancy. • Asthma or wheeziness accompanied by degrees of nausea. • Development of "sick" headaches.

COCCULUS
Cocculus orbiculatus

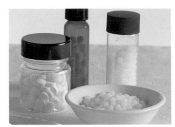

The remedy is prepared from the Indian cockle, a plant that grows along the coasts of India. It profoundly affects the nervous system and can strengthen a weakened and exhausted system. Because it can also cure nausea and dizziness, it is considered an important remedy for all kinds of travel sickness, whether on a boat, plane or in a car.

n o t e s • Nausea, vomiting, and dizziness, as in travel sickness.
• Exhaustion and nervous stress, perhaps due to lack of sleep.

DROSERA
Drosera rotundifolia

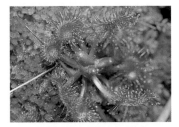

Drosera is a remedy prepared from an extraordinary insectivorous plant, the round-leaved sundew. The plants are often called "flypapers" because the leaves are tipped with sticky glands. The insect prey gets more embroiled the more it struggles, and is finally dissolved. Drosera affects the respiratory system and is an important cough remedy.

n o t e s • Deep, barking coughs.
• Prolonged and incessant coughs returning in periodic fits or spasms.
• The cough may result in retching.

EUPATORIUM
Eupatorium perfoliatum

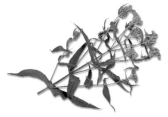

Eupatorium is a North American herb found growing in marshy places. It is used as a herb as a flu remedy, to lower fevers and even relieve congestion and constipation, as well as boosting the immune system. Its common name, boneset, gives a clue to its homeopathic use. Whatever the other symptoms, the bones usually do ache.

n o t e s • Flu-like symptoms, with aching all over, but pains that seem to have lodged deep in the bones.
• There may be a painful cough.

EUPHRASIA
Euphrasia officinalis

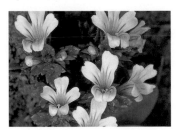

Also known as eyebright, Euphrasia has long been known as a remedy with a specific application to the eyes. It is a very pretty little meadow plant, much used in wild flower plantings, with colourful flowers that open wide only when there is direct sunshine.

n o t e s • Eyes that are sore, red and inflamed. • The eyes water with burning tears. • In cases of hay fever, the symptoms are sneezing, itching and a runny nose, but for most the eyes are most usually affected.

FERRUM PHOS
Ferrum phosphoricum

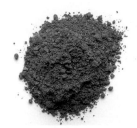

Iron phosphate, from which Ferrum phos is prepared, is a highly valued mineral that manages to balance the iron and oxygen in the blood. It is also a tissue salt and can be used actively as a tonic for anaemic patients who are beginning to feel rather weak and feeble.

n o t e s • Flu and cold symptoms that are not well defined.
• Weakness and tiredness. • General anaemia: the remedy can be very useful for women with heavy periods or during pregnancy.

GELSEMIUM
Gelsemium sempervirens

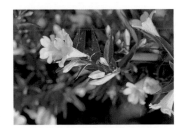

The remedy is prepared from a North American plant known as yellow jasmine. It acts specifically on the muscles, the motor nerves and the nervous system. It is also quite probably the most important acute remedy for helping to treat an attack of flu.

n o t e s • Aching, heavy muscles which will not obey the will.
• Tiredness, weakness, shivering and trembling. • Fever with sweating but little thirst. • Headaches concentrated at the back of the head.

HEPAR SULPH
Hepar sulphuris calcareum

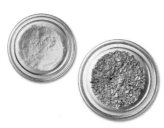

The remedy was developed by Samuel Hahnemann, the first homeopath, from calcium sulphide, which is made by heating flowers of sulphur and the lime of oyster shells together. It strongly affects the nervous system and is good in acute septic states (infected areas) and in respiratory system problems.

n o t e s • Extreme irritability and over-sensitivity. • Coldness, especially around the head. • Hoarse, dry coughs with yellow mucus, croup. • Evidence of unusually heavy sweating.

HYPERICUM
Hypericum perforatum

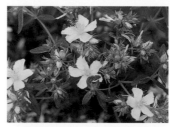

Prepared from the herb St John's Wort, Hypericum is primarily an injury remedy. It is particularly effective on any areas that have an abundant supply of sensitive nerves. They include the fingers, toes, lips, ears, eyes, and the coccyx at the base of the spine. Apply Hypericum instead of Arnica for bruising in such sensitive areas, although Arnica may work perfectly well if Hypericum is not available.

n o t e s • Pains are often felt suddenly shooting up the limbs, travelling along the tracks of the nerves.

IGNATIA
Ignatia amara

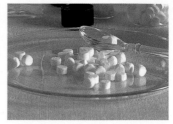

Ignatia is prepared from the seeds of a tree, the St Ignatius bean, which grows in South-east Asia. It is well known as a major "grief" remedy, and it can strongly affect the emotions.

n o t e s • Sadness and grief following emotional loss. • Sudden changeable moods: tears following laughter, or hysteria. • Suppressed emotions, when the tears will not flow. • Pronounced bouts of sighing following a period of emotional unhappiness, particularly anxiety, fear or grief.

KALI BICH
Kali bichromicum

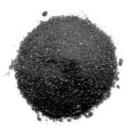

The source of Kali bichromicum, potassium dichromate, is a chemical compound involved in many industrial processes which include dyeing, printing and photography. It especially affects the mucous membranes of the air passages, and is an important sinusitis remedy.

n o t e s • Highly unpleasant thick, strong, lumpy green discharges from the nasal passages or mouth. • Headaches in small spots as a result of catarrh. • Dry cough accompanied by sticky, yellow-green mucus.

LACHESIS
Lachesis muta

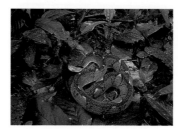

Lachesis is prepared from the venom of the bushmaster snake which is native to South America. It is a chronic remedy best left to expert, professional homeopaths, but it does have an acute use when treating sore throats and also various menstrual problems.

n o t e s • Sore throats, much worse on the left side. • Painful throats where liquids are more difficult to swallow than solids. • Menstrual pains and tension improve when the flow starts. • Hot flushes around the menopause.

LEDUM
Ledum palustre

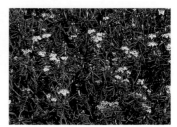

The small shrub known as marsh tea, from which Ledum is derived, grows in boggy places across the cold wastes of the Northern Hemisphere. It is primarily a first-aid injury remedy when cold rather than warmth soon brings welcome, soothing relief.

n o t e s • Puncture wounds from nails or splinters, bites and stings, when pain is eased by cold compresses. • Wounds that look puffy and feel cold. • Injuries to the eye which looks cold, puffy and bloodshot.

LYCOPODIUM
Lycopodium clavatum

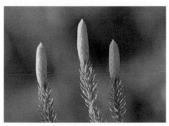

This remedy is prepared from the spores of club moss, a strange prostrate plant which likes to grow on heaths. It is generally prescribed constitutionally for aiding chronic conditions but it can also be very helpful for digestive problems and sometimes even acute sore throats.

n o t e s • Conditions which are worse on the right side, or move from the right to the left side of the body.
• Flatulence and pain in the abdomen or stomach. • Problem is aggravated by gassy foods such as beans.

CANTHARIS
Lytta vesicatoria

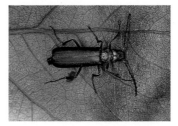

Cantharis is one of a few homeopathic remedies prepared from insects. It is derived from an iridescent green beetle which is commonly called Spanish fly. It is also known as the blister beetle because it is actually a major irritant if handled. It has an affinity with the urinary tract.

n o t e s • Cystitis – where there are highly uncomfortable, intense, burning-pains on urinating. • Evidence of burns or burning pains generally, as you would normally expect to get following sunburn, or burns from a hot pan.

MAG PHOS
Magnesia phosphorica

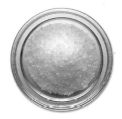

Magnesia phosphorica is one of the 12 tissue salts, as well as being a proven remedy. It is well known that it works directly in helping to ease tension in the nerves as well as in the muscles. It can therefore be considered as a very effective painkiller.

n o t e s • Violent, cramping and spasmodic pains, often in the abdominal area. • Pains better for warmth, gentle massage and doubling up.
• Can help with colic, period pains, sciatica, toothache and earache.

CHAMOMILLA
Matricaria chamomilla

Chamomile is a member of the daisy family. It strongly affects the nervous system. It is one of the most important medicines for the treatment of children: Aconite, Belladonna and Chamomilla are together known as the "ABC" remedies.

n o t e s • Bad temper and irritability.
• Teething problems in angry babies.
• In cases of colic, the stools are usually offensive, slimy and green.
• Extreme sensitivity to pain.
• The child's temper is considerably improved on being rocked or carried.

MERCURIUS
Mercurius solubilis

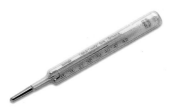

The name of this remedy is sometimes abbreviated to Merc sol. It is prepared from the liquid metal mercury. It is used in acute septic states (infected areas) where the glands and their secretions are particularly affected.

n o t e s • Swollen and tender glands.
• Profuse sweating and increased thirst. • Breath, sweat and secretions can be offensive. • The tongue looks flabby, yellow and coated.
• Fevers blow hot and cold.
• Irritability and restlessness.

PHOSPHORUS
Phosphorus

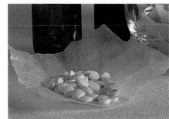

Phosphorus is an important constituent of the body, particularly of the bones. It can be useful in acute situations. These include digestive problems, with immediate vomiting once the food is warmed in the stomach, and constant diarrhoea. Phosphorus can also help aid minor haemorrhages (i.e. nosebleeds). It also relieves the "spacey" feeling that lingers too long after an anaesthetic.

n o t e s • Suits people who are lively, open and friendly, but who are also occasionally nervous and anxious.

PHYTOLACCA
Phytolacca decandra

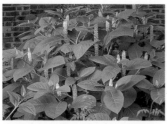

Phytolacca or poke-root is a well-known erect, unpleasant smelling plant that grows across the Northern Hemisphere, and also in South America. It is a glandular remedy that particularly affects the tonsils, and also the mammary glands. It is reckoned that Phytolacca is probably the most important remedy for helping in the treatment of mastitis.

n o t e s • Sore throats that look dark and angry. • Sore throats in which the pain feels like a hot ball. • Swollen, tender breasts with cracked nipples.

PULSATILLA
Pulsatilla nigricans

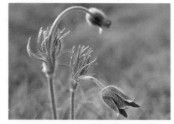

Pulsatilla is one of the most useful of acute remedies, as well as being a very important constitutional one. The remedy comes from the pasque flower and is also known as the weathercock remedy because it suits people whose moods and symptoms are constantly changing. For this reason, it is considered a wonderful remedy for small children.

n o t e s • Tendency to be weepy and clingy. • Suits people with gentle, sympathetic natures.• Yellow-green discharge from the eyes or nose.

RHUS TOX
Rhus toxicodendron

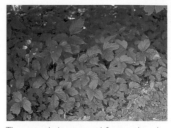

The remedy is prepared from poison ivy, native to North America. Its main use is in sprains, strains and swollen joints, but because of its itchy, rashy picture it can be a good remedy for illnesses such as chickenpox or shingles. It is also a useful remedy for acute rheumatism.

n o t e s • Extreme restlessness with a red, itchy rash. • Stiffness in the joints, which is eased by gentle motion. • The symptoms are far better for warmth, and considerably worse with cold, damp and over-exertion.

RUTA
Ruta graveolens

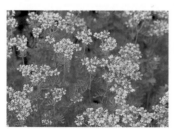

Ruta, or rue, is a much valued, highly attractive garden plant with blue-green leaves. It is also an ancient herbal remedy that has been often called the herb of grace. It acts particularly well on the joints, tendons, cartilages and periosteum (the membrane that covers the bones). It also has an affinity with the eyes.

n o t e s • Bruises to the bones. • Strains to the joints and connecting tissue, especially to the ankles and wrists. • The symptoms are worse for cold and damp and better for warmth.

SEPIA
Sepia officinalis

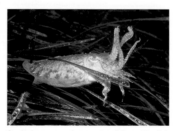

Sepia is a remedy prepared from the ink of the squid or cuttlefish. Normally its use should be left to the professional homeopath as it has a "big" picture (i.e. it can be used in many circumstances), but because of its affinity with the female reproductive system it can be helpful in some menstrual problems.

n o t e s • Suits tired, depressed, emotionally withdrawn people. • Morning sickness in pregnancy, which is worse for the smell of food. • Hot flushes during the menopause.

SILICA
Silicea

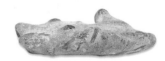

Silica is a mineral derived from flint. It is one of the 12 tissue salts, and its presence in the body aids the vital elimination of toxins. It can be used acutely in septic (infected) conditions to strengthen the body's resistance to continual infection, and also to help expel any foreign bodies such as splinters.

n o t e s • Suitable for symptoms that are slow to heal, or for people who feel the cold, or who lack stamina or vitality. • Small-scale infections that seem to be turning septic rather than healing.

SPONGIA
Spongia tosta

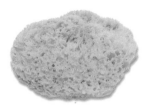

Spongia, as its name clearly indicates, is a remedy which is prepared from the lightly roasted skeleton part of the marine sponge. It actually works very well on the respiratory tract, and it is now generally considered to be one of homeopathy's major cough remedies. It is actually a significant and indeed important aid or remedy when it comes to treating croup in young children.

notes • Dry spasmodic cough.
• The cough sounds like a saw being pulled through wood.

NUX VOMICA
Strychnos nux vomica

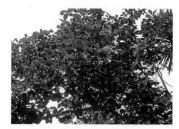

Nux vomica is prepared from the seeds of the poison nut tree of South-east Asia. It is a remedy that has many uses in both chronic and acute situations, and it is known to be very useful when the digestive system is involved.

notes • Nausea or vomiting after a rich meal, when the food remains undigested like a load in the stomach.
• A feeling that if only you could vomit you would feel better. • An urge to pass a stool, but with unsatisfactory results. • Heartburn.

SYMPHYTUM
Symphytum officinale

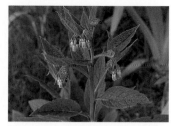

The remedy is easily prepared from the common herb comfrey. It is also called knitbone, which indicates its main use in promoting the healing of broken bones. Use the remedy daily for several weeks after the bone has been set. Symphytum can also be used for many injuries to the eyeball such as, for example, getting a tennis ball directly in the eye.

notes • Speeds up the knitting or fusing together of broken bones.
• Injuries to the eyeball, such as being hit by a hard object.

VALERIAN
Valeriana officinalis

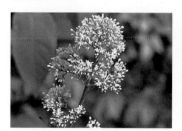

Valerian is a well-known herb whose overuse in the 19th century caused insomnia and over-taxation of the nervous system to the point of hysteria. Because of the principle "like cures like", very tiny doses such as those used in homeopathy can cure these very same problems. Valerian is an important remedy for sleeplessness. Take one pill about one hour before bedtime. You should soon notice the improvement.

notes • Especially useful when the mind feels like a "hamster on a wheel".

VERBASCUM
Verbascum thapsus

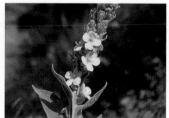

Verbascum is prepared from the great mullein, a common wayside herb. It is a highly regarded garden plant sending up marvellous stems. Homeopathically it is associated with earaches, and it is best used as an oil. The remedy is especially helpful for children, who tend to suffer from ear infections more often than adults. Place a few drops of the oil on a warmed teaspoon and gently insert into the ear, with the child lying on one side.

notes • Earaches of all kinds, both in children and adults.

VIBURNUM OPULUS
Viburnum opulus

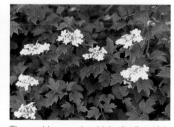

The guelder rose is widely distributed in woods and damp places throughout northern Europe and the US. It is a valued garden plant, especially in the form 'Roseum' which has large white flowers, giving rise to its common name, the snowball tree. It is also known as cramp bark and the homeopathic remedy, which is prepared from the bark, can be very helpful for period pains as well as for spasmodic cramps.

notes • For aiding the treatment of severe cramping and muscle spasms.

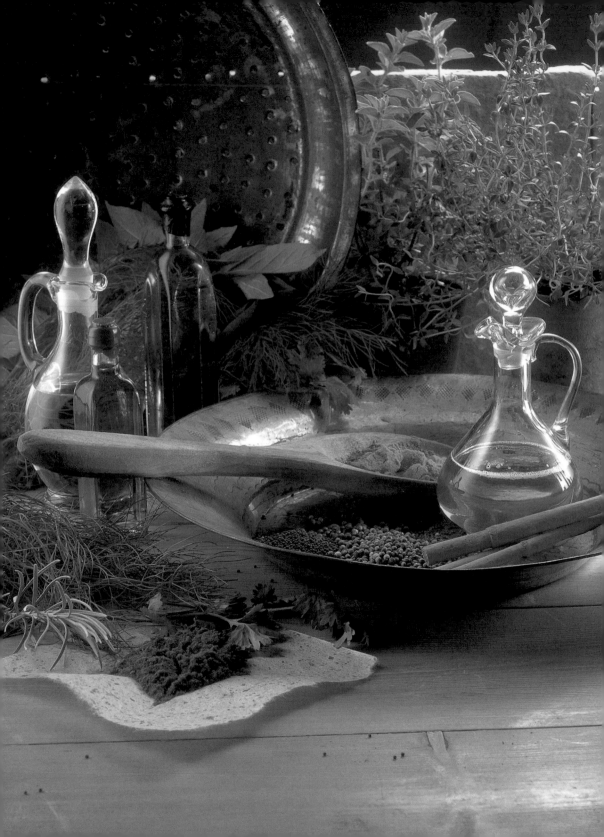

ayurveda
ayurveda

ayurveda

Ayurveda is acknowledged as the traditional healing system of India. Thousands of years old, it has influenced many other healing systems around the world. In fact, it was already established before the births of Buddha and Christ, and some biblical stories clearly reflect the wisdom of the ancient Ayurvedic teachings.

There are many different branches to Ayurveda because it covers so many aspects of health and healing. They have been touched upon in the following pages, but the main emphasis is on diet and lifestyle, specifically tailored to the modern life.

Ayurvedic medicine is founded on the belief that all diseases stem from the digestive system and are caused either by poor digestion of food, which is the body's major source of nourishment, or by following an improper diet for your dosha (nature). Here you will find basic advice about suitable diets, as well as information about supportive treatments, including massage, exercise, colour, crystals, herbs and spices. There is also a list of common ailments that can be treated.

The following basic Ayurvedic approach will help you to develop some simple ways to keep yourself balanced in these days of increasing worry and stress. Identify your dosha, learn how to live in accordance with your own true nature, and discover how you can at last begin to heal your vikruti (current emotional, physical or mental health conditions) with the use of the best basic Ayurvedic methods.

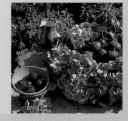

what is ayurveda?

It may be little known – and remarkably few people seem to have heard of it – but Ayurveda is a highly respected, highly revered ancient form of learning which has an amazing amount to teach us. It brings peace of body and mind, important ways of seeing the world and your own place in the scheme of things, and highly practical, sensible ideas when it comes to medicine, diet and ways of staying calm and relaxed.

THE ORIGINS OF AYURVEDA

The origins of Ayurveda are uncertain. It is recounted that thousands of years ago, men of wisdom or rishis (meaning seers) as they are known in India, were saddened by the suffering of humanity. They knew that ill health and short lives allowed man little time to consider his spirituality and to commune with the divine – with God.

In the Himalayan mountains they prayed hard and meditated together, calling upon God to help them to relieve the plight of man, and God felt moved by compassion and gave them the essential teachings that would enlighten them in the ways of healing illness, and thereby alleviate and remove all suffering on the earth.

It is believed that these teachings are the Vedas, although this cannot be proven, due to the lack of historical records. A book called the *Atharva Veda* was one of the first detailed accounts of the system. From this, and perhaps other ancient writings, came

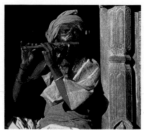

Indian sadhus, like the one shown here, tend to live a nomadic life, renouncing worldly goods, and devoting themselves to prayer.

the beginnings of Ayurvedic medicine, which has developed, changed and absorbed many other influences over hundreds of years to become what it is today. Due to the invasions of India over the years, and the subsequent suppression of many original Indian ways of life, several ancient texts have been lost or even destroyed, but enough have survived to ensure the active continuation of these highly valued, greatly respected teachings.

Ayurveda is now acknowledged as the traditional healing system of India. It comes from two Sanskrit words, *ayur*, meaning "life", and *veda*, meaning "knowing", and can be interpreted as meaning the "science of life". The oldest healing system to remain intact, it is very comprehensive and has influenced many healing systems around the world.

Ayurveda travelled out of India and influenced many other countries with its ageless wisdom about living in the light of truth.

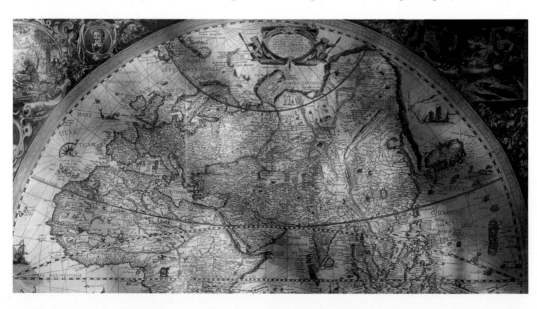

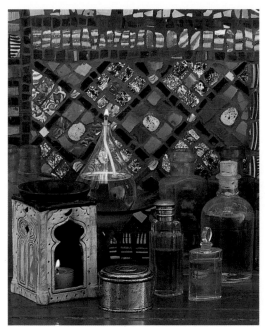

The influence of Ayurveda has spread far and wide. This is reflected in the different oils that are used. Many are made from plants that are found all over the world, not just India.

THE INFLUENCE OF AYURVEDA

For centuries after the end of the Vedic era, Ayurvedic medicine developed into a comprehensive healing system. Its philosophy and techniques soon spread far and wide to China, Arabia, Persia and Greece, gradually influencing Middle Eastern, Greek and Chinese methods of healing. It is well known that Ayurvedic practitioners reached the ancient city of Athens, and it can be noted that the traditional Greek folk medicine, based upon the bodily humours (characteristics), is significantly similar to Ayurveda. In turn, Greek medicine strongly influenced the subsequent development of what we call traditional or orthodox Western medicine. However, it is much too difficult to say exactly how much or to what degree the medical philosophy of Ayurveda was indeed influential, or even how much Ayurveda influenced current techniques.

Greek and European Medicine

The five elements in Chinese medicine appear to have come from Ayurveda. It is documented that the Indian medical system was brought to China by Indian Buddhist missionaries, many of whom were skilled Ayurvedic practitioners. The missionaries also travelled to South east Asia and Tibet, influencing the people of these lands. Tibetan medicine, for example, is an intricate mix of Ayurvedic practices and philosophy with a Tibetan Buddhist and shamanic influence.

WHAT IS AYURVEDIC MEDICINE?

The main aim of Ayurvedic medicine (which is only one branch of Ayurveda) is to improve health and longevity, leaving the individual free to contemplate matters of the spirit and to follow a spiritual path. This does not mean that you have to be spiritual or religious to benefit from Ayurvedic medicine; the system is very practical in its applications and deals with all kinds of health problems, without spirituality ever being mentioned. Its main focus is nutrition, supported primarily by the use of herbs, massage and aromatic oils, but there are many complementary branches as well.

Ayurvedic philosophy encourages those who practise it to eat the fruits and seeds of the earth, rather than take the life of animals. Since some animal products have in fact been included in this introductory guide, they should only ever be used in strict moderation. Let common sense and sensitivity be your guide.

The branches of Ayurvedic medicine include specific diets, surgery, jyotish (Vedic astrology), psychiatry and pancha karma (cleansing and detoxifying techniques). Yoga is not a branch of Ayurveda, but since it shares the same roots you will find that the two are often practised together. Yoga includes meditation, mantras (prayer chants), yantras (contemplation of geometric visual patterns) and hatha yoga (practices for bringing great harmony to the spirit, mind and body).

If you are actually much more interested in the many spiritual aspects of Ayurvedic teachings, then it is strongly recommended that you think very seriously about taking up yoga so that it becomes a regular part of your life.

Most people clearly benefit from meditation or yoga, which can help to illuminate the pathway to inner relaxation and peace.

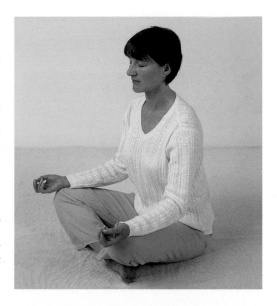

the doshas
Instead of using modern psychology to group people into types, try using the ancient doshas. They pinpoint and identify three basic types of people, which in turn helps you to a greater self-awareness and to an appreciation of others. The doshas are also excellent ways of helping you to fine-tune and regulate your lifestyle, bringing greater peace and well-being. The doshas are not just terms, they are ways of actively improving your life.

THE SEASONS

There are three doshas (basic types of people, in terms of constitution) – vata, pitta and kapha. They are influenced by the rhythms of nature, seasonal change and the time of year. Autumn is a time of change when leaves turn brown and dry; vata is highest in the autumn and early winter, and at times of dry, cold and windy weather. Pitta is highest in late spring, throughout the summer and during times of heat and humidity. Kapha is highest in the winter months and during early spring, when the weather is frequently still cold and damp.

In Ayurvedic theory, the progress of a disease goes through several stages. There is accumulation (when it is increasing), followed by aggravation (when it is at its highest point and can cause problems). There is also decrease (when it is lessening) and a neutral time when it is passive (neither decreasing nor increasing). Use the questionnaire later in this chapter to discover your dosha, and see whether it is vata, pitta or kapha. People who are single types can refer to the dosha that scores the highest points on their questionnaire. Dual doshic types should vary their lifestyle to suit the seasonal changes, as shown in the dual doshas section.

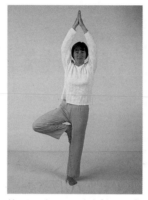

Yoga can be a very helpful way of balancing both the body and mind. After a few classes you are free to practise by yourself.

YOUR BODY TYPE

This section clearly outlines how you can identify your dosha or body type. Dosha means "that which tends to go out of balance easily." Your dosha is in fact your bio-type or prakruti ("nature"). You are made up of a mixture of the five elements – ether, wind, fire, water and earth, and will display certain recognizable characteristics depending on your personality and nature.

As well as your prakruti, you may also have a vikruti, which is your current state of mental or physical health. This develops throughout your life and may actually differ from your prakruti. It is important that you treat your vikruti first (how you are now), then go back to living with your prakruti. For example, you may have developed arthritis or back trouble over a long period, or you may be suffering from a cold or skin rash which lasts a few days. Once you have have cleared your condition, maintain your prakruti using a preventative treatment, such as diet, massage, oils, colours and scents.

Levels of vata increase in the autumn when the weather is changeable. Surrounding yourself with flowers helps you relax.

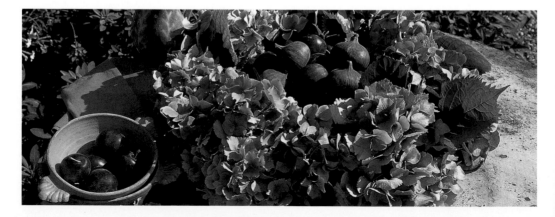

Apart from the three single doshas, there are four combinations, making a total of seven differing constitutional types: vata, pitta, kapha, vata/pitta (or pitta/vata), pitta/kapha (or kapha/pitta), kapha/vata (or vata/kapha), and vata/pitta/kapha. These may be either out of balance or in a state of balance.

To discover your prakruti and vikruti, answer the questionnaire twice. Also ask other people who know you well to fill out the questionnaire for you, to give you as clear a picture of yourself as possible. The first time you fill out the questionnaire, you should concentrate upon your current condition – your vikruti – recording your answers based upon your present and recent health history.

You can discover your prakruti by answering the questionnaire a second time, this time with answers based upon your entire lifetime. Fill out the questionnaire with your complete history in mind. This will give you a better idea about the difference between your vikruti and your prakruti. Once the answers to the questionnaire have revealed both your vikruti and your prakruti (they may be the same, which is fine), the information here can be used to treat both. Follow whichever dosha scores most highly (vata, pitta or kapha).

ELEMENTAL ENERGIES

The elements are very important in Ayurveda. They descend from space (ether), down to air. Air descends into the fire element. Fire falls into the water element and water to earth, so that we move from the most rarefied elements (ether), to the most dense (earth). With this in mind, you will notice that the chart below follows a descending pattern of ether and air (vata), fire and water (pitta) and water and earth (kapha). Vata is a mixture of ether and air and is often translated as "wind". In the creation story of Ayurveda, vata leads the other doshas, because its combination of air and ether is actually the most rarefied. The elements move from the most refined down to the most dense. Consequently, if a vata is out of balance, the end result will be that the others will be out of balance as well.

Your age and the season of the year will also have an influence upon your doshic type. From childhood up to the teenage years you are influenced by kapha; from your teens to the age of 50 or 60 you tend to come under the pitta influence, and from 50 to 60 onwards you enter the vata phase of life.

Each dosha has a particular energetic principle which influences responses within the body. Everyone has all three doshas to an extent, but it is the ratio between each that is important, and that creates your individuality. Each dosha plays an important role in this equation and balancing act. For example, movement (vata) without the stability of kapha would simply end up in chaos, and the inactivity of kapha without activity and movement would quickly result in stagnation.

A kapha type (water and earth) will be intuitive, sensitive and will dislike change but will be good at holding things together.

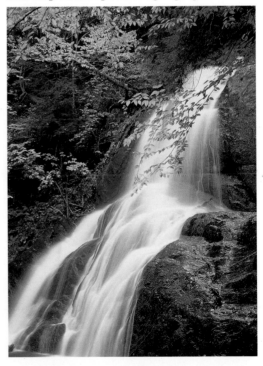

Element	Dosha	Cosmic link	Principle	Influence
ether/air	vata	wind	change	activity/movement
fire/water	pitta	sun	conversion	metabolism/transformation
water/earth	kapha	moon	inertia	cohesion

You and Your Dosha

Working out exactly which dosha type you are is easily done, but before tackling the questionnaire on the opposite page, read the following notes very carefully. They put this huge wealth of information, and its references to skin types, lifestyle, and speech, into an objective framework, giving you a clearer perspective, helping you understand precisely what are called your humoral factors.

WHICH TYPE ARE YOU?

The questionnaire opposite is designed to help you to assess your basic ratio of humoral factors. From this you can determine which diet, colours, exercise routines, crystals, oils and scents are most likely to suit you. By referring to the sections on which you score the most points, you will identify whether you are a vata, pitta or kapha dosha, or what is called a combination type. Read the questions and, to discover your prakruti, tick those descriptions which apply to you in general terms. Allocate two ticks to the statement that you think is most applicable to you; use one tick for a description that could also possibly apply, but if a particular description does not apply to you, then leave it unticked.

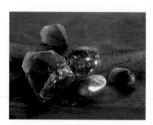

Gems are used in Ayurveda only with a prescription from a jyotish (Vedic or Hindu astrologer), or from an Ayurvedic physician.

Revealing your Vikruti

As has already been explained, your current condition, or vikruti, may not be the same as your underlying constitution, or prakruti. If you wish to discover whether or not this is the case, go through the questions a second time, this time using crosses instead of ticks. To reveal your vikruti, answer the questions according to how you have been feeling in the more recent past, and how the descriptions relate to your current health or condition, including any illnesses or other changes, no matter how subtle, that you are currently experiencing.

When you are answering the questions, do make sure that you clearly focus either on your prakruti (your general state throughout life – ticks), or on your vikruti (current or recent state – crosses). To avoid any possible confusion, make sure that you finish with one set of answers before you start attempting to fill out and assess the questionnaire for a second time.

If you wish, you can answer the questionnaire a third time, separating questions about the mind from questions about the body. Use circles and squares to record your answers. This will indicate whether your body and mind are the same dosha. If they are different, follow the dietary advice for the mind. For example, if you have a kapha body and a pitta mind, follow the kapha eating and exercise plan, including the massage technique, and ensure that you have soothing colours and a calm environment.

"Vata", "Pitta", and "Kapha"

Following the questionnaire are three sections headed "Vata", "Pitta" and "Kapha". Having discovered your vikruti (condition) or prakruti (constitution), turn to the pages relevant to your predominant dosha for detailed advice on reducing any excess

Vatas need to learn how to be still because they tend to suffer from energy depletion, having the least amount of stamina.

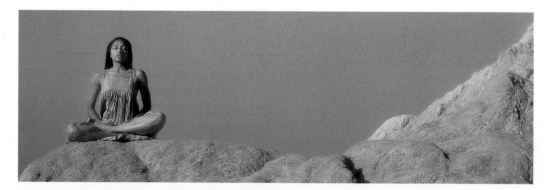

(vikruti), or to see how you can maintain your true character (prakruti). When referring to the various sections, do please read the information very carefully before you begin to put it into practice. Please also note that when using Ayurvedic medicinal herbs, you should take them only for as long as you are experiencing any obvious symptoms. You must check that the herbs are suited to your basic doshic needs; do this quite frequently, monitoring yourself even on a weekly basis.

When you begin to use any of the Ayurvedic prescriptions and techniques, do not be tempted to try and elaborate on them. This will do far more harm than good. The effect of the prescriptions lies in the ratio of the individual ingredients. Change this even in the subtlest way and all the good work may well be undone. Ayurveda is extremely complex and precise. For example, there are lengthy guidelines about the specific crystals that may be used to make a crystal infusion for each individual dosha. It is advisable that you do not make other infusions unless you are qualified or highly experienced; since crystals and gems can have a very powerful effect.

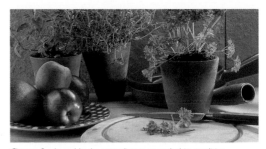

Choose foods and herbs according to your doshic condition.

Discover your Dosha

Mark the questionnaire with either a √ (= your general constitution – prakruti) or x (= your current or recent state – vikruti).

	Vata	Pitta	Kapha
HEIGHT	Very short, or tall and thin	Medium	Tall or short and sturdy
MUSCULATURE	Thin, prominent tendons	Medium/firm	Plentiful/solid
BODILY FRAME	Light, narrow	Medium frame	Large/broad
WEIGHT	Light, hard to gain	Medium weight	Heavy, gains easily
SWEAT	Minimal	Profuse, especially when hot	Moderate
SKIN	Dry, cold	Soft, warm	Moist, cool, possibly oily
COMPLEXION	Darkish	Fair, pink, red, freckles	Pale, white
HAIR AMOUNT	Average amount	Early thinning and greying	Plentiful
TYPE OF HAIR	Dry, thin, dark, coarse	Fine, soft, red, fair	Thick, lustrous, brown
SIZE OF EYES	Small, narrow or sunken	Average	Large, prominent
TYPE OF EYES	Dark brown or grey, dull	Blue/grey/hazel, intense	Blue, brown, attractive
TEETH AND GUMS	Protruding, receding gums	Yellowish, gums bleed	White teeth, strong gums
SIZE OF TEETH	Small or large, irregular	Average	Large
PHYSICAL ACTIVITY	Moves quickly, active	Moderate pace, average	Slow pace, steady
ENDURANCE	Low	Good	Very good
STRENGTH	Poor	Good	Very good
TEMPERATURE	Dislikes cold, likes warmth	Likes coolness	Aversion to cool and damp
STOOLS	Tendency to constipation	Tendency to loose stools	Plentiful, slow elimination
LIFESTYLE	Variable, erratic	Busy, tends to achieve a lot	Steady, can skip meals
SLEEP	Light, interrupted, fitful	Sound, short	Deep, likes plenty
EMOTIONAL TENDENCY	Fearful, anxious, insecure	Fiery, angry, judgemental	Greedy, possessive
MENTAL ACTIVITY	Restless, lots of ideas	Sharp, precise, logical	Calm, steady, stable
MEMORY	Good recent memory	Sharp, generally good	Good long term
REACTION TO STRESS	Excites very easily	Quick temper	Not easily irritated
WORK	Creative	Intellectual	Caring
MOODS	Change quickly	Change slowly	Generally steady
SPEECH	Fast	Clear, sharp, precise	Deep, slow
RESTING PULSE			
WOMEN	Above 80	70-80	Below 70
MEN	Above 70	60-70	Below 60
Totals: *Please add up*	**Vata**	**Pitta**	**Kapha**

vata

Vata types are known to be rather restless, cool people, who certainly notice the cold. When you have excess levels of vata, fear, depression and nervousness become quite marked, significant traits, and with repressed emotions comes a definite weakening of the immune system. However, by adopting the appropriate lifestyle, and making one or two changes, you will create a better balance within yourself, and find that you achieve much more.

The vata body type is usually thin and narrow. Vatas do not gain weight easily and are often restless by nature, especially when they are busy and active. They have dry hair and cool skin and a tendency to feel the cold. Their levels of energy are erratic, and they have to be very careful not to exhaust themselves, leading to inconsistency. They may find it quite hard to relax, which can lead to an overactive mind and insomnia.

Vata symptoms will be changeable, being cold by nature and therefore worse in cold weather. Any pain will worsen during change. Vata people can suffer from wind, low back pain, arthritis and nerve disorders. Vata types, because of their individual restless nature, certainly require a regular intake of nourishment, and they should sit down to eat or drink at regular times. Careful exercise should always be taken in moderation, clearly maintaining a gentle, regular, well-worked out routine that will help to keep the mind focused, and in perfect harmony with the body.

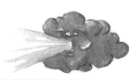

Vata people should try to eat warming foods which are earthy and sweet, with the emphasis upon cooked foods, such as a bowl of dhal, rather than salads.

Elements: ether and air.
Climate: dry and cold.
Principle: movement.
Emotions: fearful, anxious, apprehensive, sensitive, timid, lacking confidence, slightly nervous, changeable.
Systems most affected by excess vata: the nervous system and also the colon.
Symptoms of excess vata: flatulence, back pain, problems with circulation, dry skin, outbreaks of arthritis, constipation, and nerve disorders.

In summer the vata quickly begins to accumulate as the heat of the sun begins to dry everything out. The best way to stop your skin from drying out too, so keeping it gently moist, is to use a top quality natural cream.

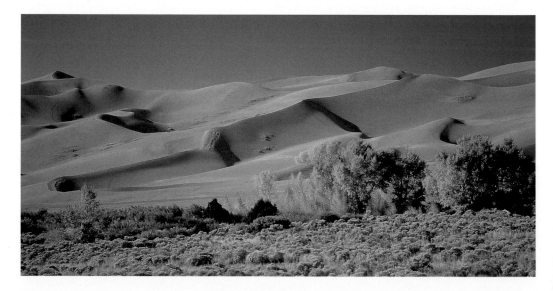

DIETARY TIPS

Vata people must always be quite careful, but not to the point that cooking suddenly becomes something of a difficult problem. The easy-to-follow, basic guidelines are as follows.

You must avoid all kinds of fried foods, no matter how tempting, and you should eat at regular intervals. Irregular huge meals are to be avoided at all costs. To reduce any excess vata, then follow the vata diet and recommendations in your eating and living plan. Always attempt to avoid any foods and other items that are not listed, as far as is possible. If animal products are a part of your diet, they should be used strictly in moderation.

HERBS AND SPICES

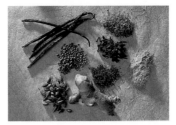

Almond essence, asafoetida (hing), basil leaves, bay leaves, cardamom pods, coriander (cilantro), fennel, fresh ginger, marjoram, mint, nutmeg, oregano, paprika, parsley, peppermint, spearmint, tarragon, thyme, turmeric and vanilla.

GRAINS AND SEEDS

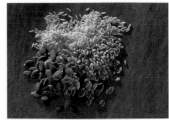

Oats (cooked), pumpkin seeds, quinoa, rice (this includes all kinds and varieties), sesame seeds, sprouted wheat bread, sunflower seeds and wheat.

NUTS, MEAT & FISH

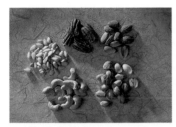

Almonds, brazil nuts, cashews, hazelnuts, macadamias, pecans, pine nuts, pistachios and walnuts. Beef, chicken, duck, eggs, sea fish, shrimps and turkey.

VEGETABLES

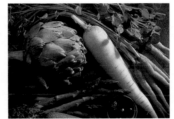

Artichokes, asparagus, beetroot, carrots, courgettes (zucchini), cucumber, daikon radish, green beans, leeks, okra, olives, onions (cooked), parsnips, pumpkins, radishes, spinach (cooked), swede (rutabagas), sweet potatoes, tomatoes (cooked), and fresh watercress.

FRUIT

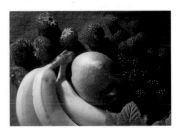

Apricots, avocados, bananas, berries, cherries, fresh coconuts, dates, fresh figs, grapefruit, grapes, lemons, limes, mangoes, melons, oranges, peaches, pineapples, rhubarb and strawberries.

DAIRY PRODUCTS

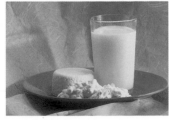

Cow's milk, cottage cheese, goat's milk, goat's' cheese and soft cheese – all are to be taken sensibly, in moderation.

COOKING OILS

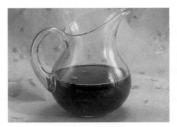

Unrefined sesame oil.

DRINKS

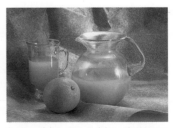

Apricot juice, carrot juice, ginger tea, grape juice, grapefruit juice, orange juice, hot dairy drinks, lemon balm tea, lemonade and peach juice.

AROMAS AND MASSAGE OILS

Vata people are unusual because they tend to benefit much more than either of the other two doshas from having a massage. Consequently they should consider massaging their feet, hands and head every morning, and have a regular massage at least once a week. The massage should become a regular, greatly appreciated part of your lifestyle.

Vata aromas are warm and sweet, and the most appropriate massage oil for the vata personality is gently warmed sesame oil. Bottles of sesame oil are widely available, and are generally of a high, well-perfumed standard. If that is impossible to obtain, any other oil (preferably virgin olive) will suffice. It can be perfumed by the addition of your favourite herb. Oil is good for vata types, and if your vata is seriously out of balance, increase the number of massages you have a week from one to as many as three. You will soon notice the enormous improvement.

When using essential oils, note they must be diluted. Do not put them directly on your skin or take them internally. In fact it is not advisable to use the same essential oil for more than two weeks; interchange your essential oils so that you do not create a toxic build-up, or overload of one fragrance. If you are pregnant or have a diagnosed medical condition, do not use any essential oil without consulting a qualified practitioner.

Warm, calming or earthy essential oils are the most suitable for vata. These include camphor (which can be an irritant, so do test yourself for sensitivity first), eucalyptus, ginger, sandalwood and jatamansi (a spikenard species from India).

vata massage

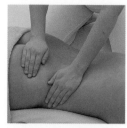

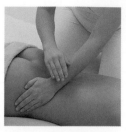

1 The correct vata massage should always be gentle.

2 Keep the actions firm, regular, soothing and relaxing.

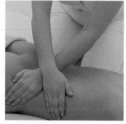

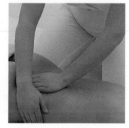

3 Use flowing, continuous stroking movements.

4 Oil and ease any areas displaying dry, tight skin.

COLOURS

Vata individuals generally benefit from most of the pastel colours, and from earthy colours that are gentle and warm to look at. They include ochres, browns and yellows.

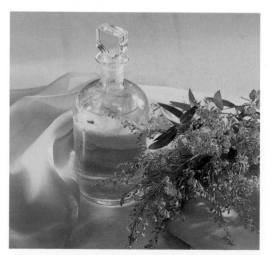

Ochre

A warm, friendly and relaxing colour, ochre is good at drawing the energy down, right through the system, helping the vata individual to feel much more solid and steady.

Brown

A solid, reliable colour, brown helps to ground the vata type, stabilizing any tendency to flightiness. It is also good at holding the emotions in place; it consolidates and aids concentration.

Yellow

A warming, enlivening colour, yellow is linked to the mind and intellect. It helps to keep the vata mentality alert by focusing the mind, and calming any rising emotions.

Making a Colour Infusion

Begin by taking a piece of thin cotton or silk. The fabric should be warm yellow in colour, and sufficiently thin to allow the light through. Next, wrap it around a small transparent (not coloured) jar filled with spring water and leave it outside in the sunlight for four hours. Finally, remove the fabric. Note, vata infusions should not be stored in the fridge, but kept at room temperature.

This infusion will encourage a sense of warmth and well-being.

GEMS AND CRYSTALS

Gems and crystals have subtle healing qualities that can be utilized in Ayurvedic medicine. Their curious, well-known powers are taken seriously by the jyotish (Vedic astrologer), who can determine which gems or crystals you will need to use, depending on the circumstances of your life chart.

Topaz is a warm stone that traditionally dispels fear, making it an ideal stone for vata because it calms high emotions and anxiety. Wear topaz whenever you want to feel confident and in control. Amethyst is an appropriate crystal to wear when you want to balance vata. It soon promotes a fine clarity of mind and thought, and will help you to radiate harmony.

There may be times when it is advisable to remove all crystals – when you find circumstances in your life are changing for the worse. This indicates that your birth chart or constitution does not require the healing qualities of a particular crystal, or that it is highlighting an area of your birth chart in a negative way. Seek expert advice on replacements.

Cleaning Crystals and Crystal Infusions

Before making a crystal infusion, it is best to cleanse your crystal. In fact, crystals that are used for infusions should ideally be cleansed before and after each use. Once you have filled a bowl with spring water, dissolve a teaspoon of sea salt in it. The crystal sits in for up to about eight hours before being rinsed.

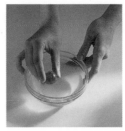 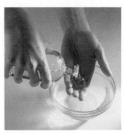

1 Place the crystal in the water and leave to stand for about four hours, or leave it overnight in the dark.

2 Rinse it in spring water, visualizing any residues that were being held in the crystal being washed away.

To make a crystal infusion, take the cleansed crystal and hold it in your hands, imagining that the crystal is full of peace and calm. Place the crystal in a clear glass bowl, cover it with spring water, and leave it in the sunlight for about four hours. Remove the crystal and bottle the spring water. You can now drink the infusion prior to any mentally demanding tasks. It will aid clarity of mind and help reduce any stress that might arise as a result of pressure. You can keep the infusion for just 24 hours, after which it should be discarded. Make sure you store the infusion away from domestic appliances and electrical equipment.

EXERCISE AND TONIC

Since vata is cold in nature it benefits from warmth and comfort. Make your own warming tonic drinks for cold windy days by combining ingredients from the vata eating plan. Be aware though that sugar weakens the immune system and vatas, with their tendency to stress (another immune suppressor), need to be particularly wary of sugary and refined foods, choosing naturally sweet-tasting foods, such as fruit, instead.

Vata people benefit from gentle, relaxing forms of exercise. Being the most easily exhausted of the various categories, they should be careful not to overdo things. Examples of suitable exercise include walking, yoga and slow swimming. In essence, it is not so much the form of exercise that you take, but rather the way in which you take it. With vata, the exercise routine should always be on the gentle side; with this in mind, vata types can undertake most sports and activities.

Yoga stretches will gradually and gently lengthen your muscles, and increase your flexibility. It has enormous all-round benefits. If you do not actively practise yoga as a form of exercise, you may well find that achieving a full or even half lotus for meditation is much too strenuous and difficult. If this is the case, do not try and force yourself. Instead, use a specifically designed meditation stool, or place some firm cushions on the floor beneath you. Push your bent knees on to the floor, then tuck your feet in towards you on the floor, forming a solid triangular base with your legs.

Fresh Ginger and Lemon Tea

This tea is remarkably quick and easy to make, and tastes absolutely delicious. It is also a marvellous tonic for a vata.

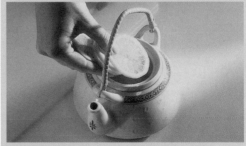

| I lemon | Spring water |
| A small slice of fresh ginger | Raw honey or fructose |

1 Wash the lemon and then cut it into thin slices, leaving the peel on. Peel the piece of fresh ginger and slice it finely.
2 Place the lemon and ginger slices in a small teapot.
3 Add boiling spring water, then stir. Finally sweeten with honey or fructose, drink and enjoy.

pitta

Pitta people are generally quite well-balanced, well-proportioned, rounded types, admired by all, but they can suddenly become passionately focused and intense. At its most extreme this tendency leads to a high degree of intolerance and irritability. Consequently pitta types should keep well away from any foods that are known to be hot and spicy, and which might inflame them, and concentrate on meals that promote their more soothing side.

The pitta body type is usually of average build and nicely proportioned. Pittas like food and have a healthy appetite. The hair is usually straight, fine and fair, though dark-haired people can also be pitta types. People with red hair will automatically have some level of pitta within their nature. Like the fire element, their temperament can be quite intense, and when it manifests itself in excess this can lead to marked intolerance.

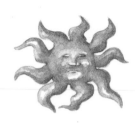

Pitta skin will have a tendency to be sensitive to the sun, and pitta types will need to be very careful how much time they spend in direct sunlight. The fiery nature of the sun will sometimes inflame the pitta person, leading to skin rashes, freckles and sunburn. Cool showers, cool environments and plenty of long cooling drinks (but not ice-cold ones) will help to alleviate any high temperatures and calm down pitta types.

People of this nature can be impatient, having highly active and alert minds. However, pitta people can also have a very good sense of humour and a warm personality.

Pitta people should always aim to eat food that is rather soothing. What they must do is avoid any foods that are considered hot and spicy. Ingredients such as fiery chillies are definitely off the menu.

Elements: fire and water.
Climate: hot and moist.
Principle: transformation.
Emotions: hate, anger, resentment, intolerance, impatience, irritability, indignation, jealousy, good humour, intelligence, alertness, open warm-heartedness.
Systems most affected by excess pitta: skin, metabolism, small intestines, eyes, liver, hair on the head.
Symptoms of excess pitta: skin disorders, acidity, sun-sensitivity, premature degrees of hair loss or loss of hair colour, outbreaks of diarrhoea.

Pitta types generally benefit from spending time away from fast, noisy, chaotic urban environments. They should seek out quiet, peaceful, well-shaded, naturally calming surroundings.

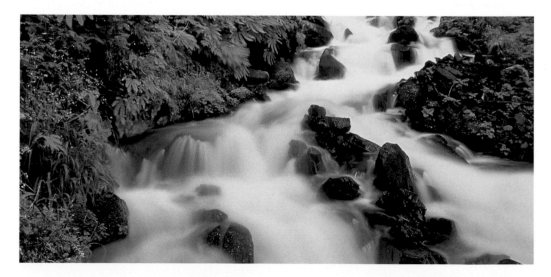

DIETARY TIPS

The pitta person should avoid all hot, spicy and sour foods, as they will aggravate this dosha; they should also avoid all fried foods. Since heated food will increase pitta within the system, pitta types should eat more raw than cooked foods. As a primarily vegetarian system, Ayurveda does not advocate the eating of animal products, especially for the pitta dosha, so although some meats and other animal products have been included in the following list, they should really be used in the strictest moderation. Let common sense always prevail.

HERBS AND SPICES

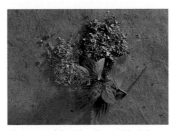

Aloe vera juice (totally avoid during a pregnancy), basil leaves, cinnamon, coriander (cilantro), cumin, dill, fennel, fresh ginger, hijiki, mint leaves, spearmint.

GRAINS AND SEEDS

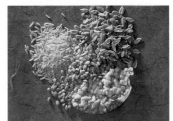

Barley, basmati rice, flax seeds, psyllium seeds, rice cakes, sunflower seeds, wheat, wheat bran, white rice.

PROTEINS

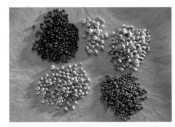

Aduki beans, black beans, black-eyed beans, chick peas (garbanzos), kidney beans, lentils (red and brown), lima beans, mung beans, pinto beans, soya beans, split peas, tempeh and tofu. Chicken, freshwater fish, rabbit, turkey.

VEGETABLES

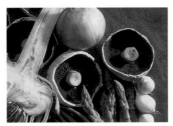

Artichokes, asparagus, broccoli, Brussels sprouts, butternut squash, cabbages, courgettes (zucchini), celery, cucumber, fennel, green beans and green peppers, Jerusalem artichokes, kale, leafy greens, leeks, lettuces, mushrooms, onions (cooked), parsnips, spinach (cooked). Eat most vegetables raw instead of cooked.

FRUIT

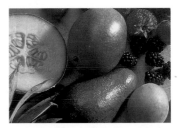

Apples, apricots, avocados, berries, cherries, dates, figs, mangoes, melons, oranges, pears, pineapples, plums, pomegranates, prunes, quinces, raisins, red grapes and watermelons. Always make sure that the fruits have fully ripened, and are very sweet and fresh.

DAIRY PRODUCTS

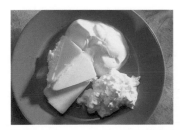

Cottage cheese, cow's milk, diluted yoghurt, ghee (clarified butter), goat's milk, mild soft cheeses and unsalted butter may all be taken but with a reasonable degree of moderation.

COOKING OILS

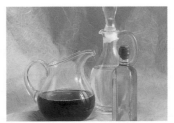

Olive oil, sunflower oil, soya and walnut oil. As with all dairy products, these oils should be used in moderation.

DRINKS

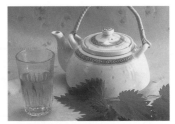

Apple juice, apricot juice, cool dairy drinks, grape juice, mango juice, mixed vegetable juice, soya milk, vegetable bouillon, elderflower tea, jasmine tea, spearmint tea and strawberry tea.

AROMAS AND MASSAGE OILS

Essential oils for pitta include honeysuckle, jasmine, sandalwood and vetiver. They must be diluted and should never be taken internally. Avoid a toxic build-up by interchanging the oils every two weeks. If you are pregnant or have a diagnosed medical condition, you must consult a qualified practitioner before attempting to use essential oils.

If possible go to an experienced masseur. They understand exactly how a massage should be given. In time you will pick up the basics and may be able to start giving others a gentle massage. The key to success is to take your time, and make sure that your partner is fully relaxed. There is no point in attempting a soft massage when they are in an agitated state, and are incapable of lying still for a couple of minutes, let alone 20. When applying the essential oils, it is important that you work with firm, consistent hand movements, totally avoiding any sudden changes of direction. Think of your hands as waves, sweeping in one long curving movement over a smooth beach. That said, do not go to the opposite extreme and be so frightened of touching or hurting the skin that you barely make any contact. The right degree of pressure is about the same as for a firm hairwash.

After the massage, do not expect to get up and rush out. That would immediately undermine all the good work. Instead, take your time, possibly even have a cat-nap, and only step back into everyday life when you are feeling absolutely ready. That way you will feel refreshed, calm and clear-headed. It also helps if you have a massage on a day that you know will be stress-free.

Pitta Massage

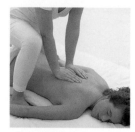
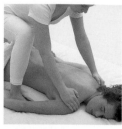

1 Start the massage in the middle of the back.

2 Use continuous, relaxing, deep, varied movements.

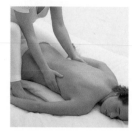
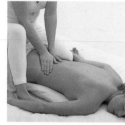

3 Be gentle on any areas of stiffness or soreness.

4 Continue with sweeping, slow movements.

COLOURS

If you are experiencing symptoms of excess pitta, such as irritability or impatience, or on occasions when you know that you are going to have a busy and active day ahead of you, balance your system by wearing natural fibres in cooling and calming colours, such as green, blue, violet or any quiet pastel shade.

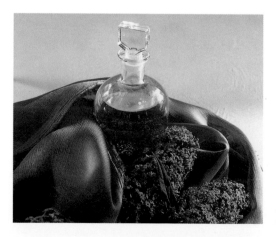

Blue

Blue is a soothing, healing colour which is ideal for the active pitta type. It is linked to spiritual consciousness and helps the pitta to remain open and calm without being over-stimulated.

Green

Green, an integral colour of the natural world, brings harmonious feelings to the pitta personality, having the ability to soothe emotions and calm passionate feelings.

Violet

Violet is a refined colour that soothes and opens the mind, and increases awareness of spiritual issues.

Making a Colour Infusion

Take a piece of thin, translucent cotton or silk in violet or light blue. Wrap it around a small transparent (not coloured) bottle or jar filled with spring water. Leave it outside in dappled sunlight, not in direct sun, for approximately six hours. Finally, remove the fabric, and drink the infusion to encourage the wonderful sensation of inner peace and harmony.

A blue colour infusion will help to clear the system of a build-up of pressure.

GEMS AND CRYSTALS

When you want to reduce excess pitta, wear pearls or a mother-of-pearl ring set in silver upon the ring finger of your right hand. Pearls have the ability to reduce inflammatory conditions, including sudden passionate, heated emotions. Ideally, natural pearls should be worn, although cultured pearls are actually quite acceptable. The most harmonious day to put on your pearls is a Monday (the moon's day) during a new moon. However, do not wear pearls when you have a kapha condition, such as a cold. The moonstone has the ability to calm emotions and is soft and cooling, being feminine in orientation. It can certainly help to pacify the pitta personality.

You can also use stones, as shown right, to make a special infusion. It involves no more than placing the stone in a glass bowl that has been topped up with spring water. The key part of the process is standing the bowl and stone outside, preferably on a night when there is a full moon and a cloudless sky. The longer you can leave it standing out the better, three hours being about the minimum period for successful results.

When you bring in the bowl, pour the special water into a clean glass and drink before breakfast. If you can make standing this bowl outside at night a regular part of your routine, then you will soon notice the difference that drinking moonstone water makes. You will feel increasingly calm, relaxed, clear-headed, stable, grounded, and above all inwardly strong. Your confidence grows and grows. You will find that other people definitely notice, and become increasingly attracted towards you. Feeling more attractive actually gives you a new lease of life.

Making a Moonstone Infusion

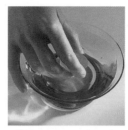

1 Take a stone specimen that has already been cleansed.

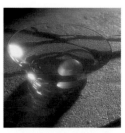

2 Leave the bowl outside to stand under a full moon.

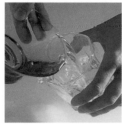

3 Remove the moonstone, and pour out the liquid.

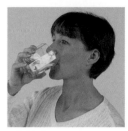

4 Drink the moonstone infusion when you wake.

Orange and Elderflower Infusion

This infusion makes a light refreshing drink, ideal in summer.

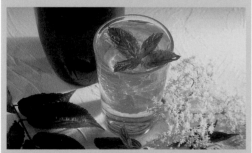

1 large sweet orange	300ml/½ pint spring water
2 heads fresh elderflower	Fructose to taste
Fresh spearmint	

1 Wash the orange in spring water. Slice and put in a jug.
2 Add elderflower heads and spearmint; pour in spring water.
3 Leave for one hour, add fructose to taste, and drink.

EXERCISE AND TONIC

Cooling drinks made from fresh fruit and vegetable juices are ideal tonics for the pitta constitution.

Pittas require a moderate amount of exercise, which should involve some element of vigour and challenge – jogging, team sports and some of the gentler martial arts which do not stress sudden, fierce, aggressive movements. Pitta exercise should not overstimulate the body, and any exercise should be kept in line with an average amount of effort and challenge. You should avoid going to such extremes that your pitta nature gets carried away and you end up overdoing it. So, for example, doubles tennis is much better for you than singles, swimming is better than squash, and gentle jogging is much better for you than sudden sprinting. In the end, though, it is not so much what you do but how you do it that is deemed important.

This orange and elderflower infusion, left, is a light and delicate alternative to a cordial. Cordials are made by boiling all the ingredients together, which is not appropriate for pitta types because of the heat required in the cooking process. In fact, a general awareness of such techniques will help you make the right decisions in all aspects of your diet. Note that drinks are just as important as anything else you might have. They contribute greatly to our overall wellbeing.

kapha

Kapha types are restless, complex, interesting contradictions. You will also find that despite being quite athletic, they actually need plenty of motivation, without which they can easily become overweight. On the plus side, they are certainly highly sensitive, but in return they do need quite a lot of sensitive handling. All in all they are thoroughly reliable, methodical people, and with that extra energy input will always stay one step ahead.

The kapha body type is well built, with a tendency to weight problems, especially if an exercise programme is not followed to keep the kapha active and moving. Kapha people are naturally athletic but they do need motivation. They are generally very sensitive and emotional, and they do require understanding otherwise they tend to turn to food as an emotional support and stabilizer. They should always ensure that what they eat is suitable for their body type. Their hair will be thick, fine and wavy, their skin soft, smooth and sensuous, and their eyes large, trusting and attractive.

Kapha people are inclined to be slow and steady, methodical and pragmatic, with a real dislike of change. They make good managers though, because they like to be reliable and available. They act like an anchor in a business because they have an innate organizing ability. Note that bright, strong, striking colours will greatly help to reduce any excess kapha, and stimulate those who are feeling slow, sluggish and dull.

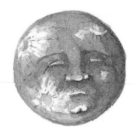

Kapha food should be light, dry, hot and stimulating. Always opt for cooked foods, such as hot and spicy vegetable curries, in preference to any kind of fresh salad.

Elements: water and earth.
Climate: cold and damp.
Principle: cohesion.
Emotions: stubbornness, greed, jealousy, possessiveness, lethargy, reliability and methodical behaviour, kindliness, motherliness.
Systems most affected by excess kapha: joints, lymphatics, body fluids and mucous membranes throughout the body.
Symptoms of excess kapha: congestion, bronchial/nasal discharge, sluggish digestion, nausea, slow mental responses, idleness, desire for sleep, excess weight, fluid retention.

Because kapha individuals have a tendency towards inertia, they need plenty of motivation. A good kick-start to the day is regular, early morning outdoor exercise, such as a brisk walk or a jog.

DIETARY TIPS

Kapha people should focus upon cooked food, but can have some salads occasionally. They should avoid fats and oils unless they are hot and spicy. Dairy products, sweet, sour and salty tastes and a high intake of wheat will also aggravate kapha. Although some meats and animal products have been included, they should always be used in moderation.

To reduce any excess levels of kapha (vikruti), or to maintain the right balance because you are a kapha dosha (prakruti), include the following items in your eating plan and try to avoid any foods that are not listed here.

HERBS AND SPICES

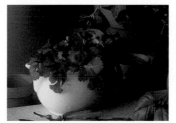

Asafoetida (hing), black or Indian pepper, chilli pepper, coriander leaves (cilantro), dry ginger, garlic, horseradish, mint leaves, mustard, parsley or any other hot spices.

GRAINS AND SEEDS

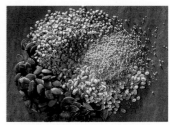

Barley, buckwheat, corn, couscous, oat bran, polenta, popcorn (plain), rye, sprouted wheat bread, toasted pumpkin seeds and occasional small quantities of toasted sunflower seeds.

BEANS AND PULSES

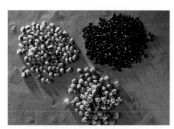

Aduki beans, black-eyed beans, chick peas (garbanzos), lima beans, pinto beans, red lentils, split peas and tempeh.

MEAT AND FISH

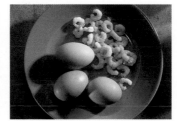

Eggs, freshwater fish, turkey, rabbit, shrimps and venison.

VEGETABLES

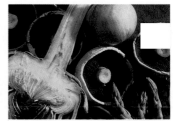

Artichokes, broccoli, Brussels sprouts, cabbage, carrots, cauliflower, celery, daikon radish, fennel, green beans, kale, leeks, lettuce, mushrooms, okra, onions, peas, peppers, radishes, spinach. Kapha vegetables should be cooked.

FRUITS

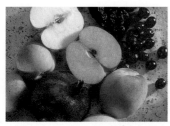

Apples, apricots, berries, cherries, peaches, pears, pomegranates and prunes.

COOKING OILS

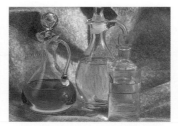

Corn, almond or sunflower oil may be used in small quantities.

DRINKS

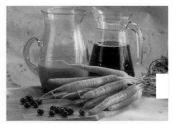

Fruit drinks should not contain sugar or additives. Recommended hot drinks include black tea, carrot juice, cranberry juice, grape juice, mango juice, mixed vegetable juice, nettle tea, passion flower tea, raspberry tea and occasional wine.

AROMAS AND MASSAGE OILS

Kapha individuals require minimal oil or none at all with massage, using instead a natural, unscented talcum powder which can be purchased from most health food stores. If an essential oil is used at all, the best ones for kapha individuals include eucalyptus, cinnamon, orange peel (since this can cause sun sensitivity, avoid strong sunlight after a massage with orange peel), ginger and myrrh. All of these oils are stimulating and it would be well advisable, after diluting approximately 7–10 drops of essential oil in 25ml/1fl oz carrier oil, to test an area of skin first to check for any possible sensitive reaction.

Unlike the sensitive gentleness of the pitta massage with its sweeping regular movements designed to relax, the kapha is actually quite fast and vigorous. You will notice that when having a massage the hands sweep over you firmly and energetically, keeping to a constant rhythm. If giving such a massage to a friend or partner, be aware that it can surprisingly be quite tiring. The aim is to kick-start and stimulate the metabolism that tends towards the sluggish.

Concentrate on the hip and groin areas to encourage lymphatic drainage, and also around the armpits to release any congestion. Finally, note as always that essential oils must be diluted and should not be taken internally. Do not to use the same essential oil for more than two weeks. If you are pregnant or have a diagnosed medical condition, do not use any essential oil without consulting a qualified practitioner. The risks are not worth taking.

Kapha Massage

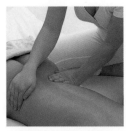

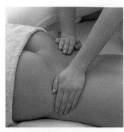

1 Kapha massage needs to fairly vigorous and stimulating.

2 Use fast movements, using talcum powder.

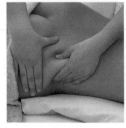

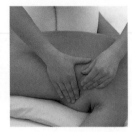

3 Use hip/groin massage to assist lymphatic drainage.

4 Another major lymph gland area is around the armpits.

COLOURS

Kapha individuals benefit from the warm and stimulating colours of the spectrum. Whenever you experience symptoms such as lethargy and sluggishness, which suggest excess kapha, or if you need to be particularly active, wear bright, invigorating, stimulating colours. You will quickly notice how effective they are, inspiring a change in your temperament.

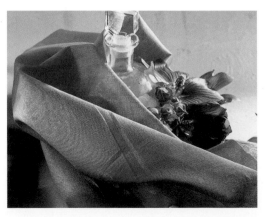

Red

Red is the colour of blood and will increase circulation as well as being energizing and positive. It should be used sparingly to avoid over-stimulation of kapha, creating excess pitta.

Orange

Orange is a warming, nourishing colour which feeds the sexual organs, and its glowing colour helps to remove congestion.

Pink

Warm, comforting pinks gently stimulate kapha into activity. Being a softer colour than red, pink may be worn without ill-effects for significantly longer periods. A highly useful colour.

Making a Colour Infusion

Take a piece of thin cotton or silk. The fabric should be a warm pink and sufficiently translucent to allow the light to penetrate. Wrap it around a transparent (not coloured) small bottle containing spring water. Stand it in full sunlight or upon a windowsill with the window open so that the light can fall naturally upon the bottle. Leave it for about four hours. Remove the fabric and drink the contents of the bottle within 24 hours.

If possible, choose a fabric which has been dyed with natural dyes.

GEMS AND CRYSTALS

Lapis lazuli is a reliably suitable, highly useful crystal with which to reduce any excess levels of kapha. Known as the heavenly stone it will quickly help kapha individuals to increase their bodily vibrations, raising them from the level of the dense and slow to a much more refined and spiritual resonance. Lapis lazuli is a quite remarkable crystal, one that is well worth seeking out.

Crystal Infusion

Cleanse your lapis lazuli prior to making an infusion. Hold the lapis in your hands for a few moments, visualizing clarity and inspiration. Take your time to get this right. The crystal should now be ready for use. Place it in a clear glass bowl and cover it with spring water. Leave it outside in the sunlight for about four hours. The brighter and sunnier the sky, the better. Next, remove the crystal, and bottle the infused spring water. You can regularly drink small amounts of it throughout the day, as required, and this will certainly ensure a continued rising of your spirits towards inspired, enlivened action.

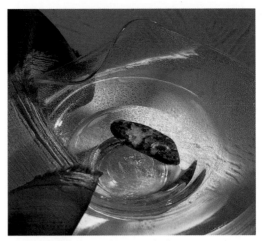

Make a lapis infusion to reduce excess kapha.

EXERCISE AND TONIC

Kapha types may well avoid this page because it suggests exercise! However, kapha people must address their natural aversion to physical activity. Exercise will make an amazing difference, cleansing excess kapha, and making valuable room for their inner beauty and radiance to shine right through.

Since kapha individuals will tend to shy away from any vigorous exercise, a certain amount of self-discipline is required. Once a regular exercise routine is established, however, the kapha type will enjoy and benefit from the enlivened and energetic feeling that all activity and exercise brings. Examples of fairly vigorous exercise well suited to the kapha type include running, fast swimming, aerobics and even fitness training. If at all unused to such exercise, start with a gentle routine, and seek guidance from an expert, qualified trainer.

It is advisable to increase the exercise level during colder spells of weather when extra stimulation is required. If this becomes a regular routine it will really push the kapha type. The benefits will soon be obvious.

Kapha people need to ensure that they have vigorous exercise, such as aerobics.

Spiced Yogi Tea

Spiced yogi tea is a delicious, warming drink which will soon help to reduce any excess kapha and is perfect for warming up cold bones on a chilly winter's day.

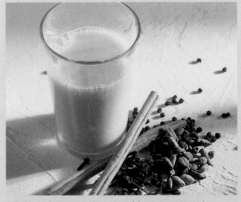

2.5ml/½ tsp dry ginger
4 whole cardamom pods
5 cloves
A pinch of black pepper or pippali (Indian long pepper)

1 large cinnamon stick
600ml/1 pint/2½ cups spring water
30ml/2tbsp goat's milk or organic soya milk

1 Mix the spices together in a saucepan.
2 Add the spring water and boil off half the liquid.
3 Turn off the heat and add the goat's milk or soya milk.
4 Stir and strain the liquid. Serve hot.

dual doshas

In all relationships, at home and work, it will make a great difference if you can try to adopt the approaches recommended for your own particular dosha. The vata dosha may well need to work at being much more reliably consistent, with the pitta dosha aiming at far greater tolerance and patience. The rather possessive kapha dosha, on the other hand, should always put extra trust and flexibility right at the top of the list.

Vata/Pitta – Pitta/Vata

If, when you answered the questionnaire in the introduction, you found that you scored twice as many points on any one type as on the other two, this means that you will predominantly be that type. For example, a score of 30 points on kapha and 5 or 10 on the others would indicate that you are a kapha type. However, if there is a closer gap with perhaps 30 points for kapha and 20 for pitta then you are classified as a kapha/pitta type. If you are such a dual type, read the following essential information.

Vata/pitta is a combination of ether/air and fire/water elements. If you belong to this dual type, refer to both the vata and the pitta eating and living plans. Choose items from the pitta plan during the spring and summer months, and during outbreaks of hot, humid weather. Follow the vata plan during the autumn and winter months, and during any cold, dry spells. For example, pungent foods aggravate pitta but can actually help to calm vata (because vata is cold), which is why the plans need to be changed in accordance with the weather, your health and a wide range of other factors. It is really quite important that you keep

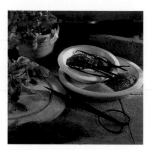

Vata/pitta – pitta/vata herbs include the different kinds of basil, coriander (cilantro), cumin seeds, fennel, mint, turmeric and vanilla pods.

a regular, accurate check on such factors, and modify your approach accordingly.

Eat your vegetables in season, and mostly cooked and flavoured with appropriate vata spices to minimize aggravation of vata and pitta. Only small amounts of bitter vegetables should be used. Among foods suitable for the vata/pitta type are broccoli, cauliflower, cucumber, endive, kale, onion (cooked), plantain, coconut, sweet oranges, apricots and other sweet fruits. Teas that are beneficial include elderflower, fennel, lemon balm and rosehip teas. Appropriate herbs and spices for vata/pitta – pitta/vata include fresh basil, caraway, cardamom, cumin, fennel, garam masala, spearmint and vanilla.

The nature of vata is change and when you are more familiar with the doshic influences that the climate has on you, you may be more flexible with the doshic recommendations. Remember, though, that you are influenced by everything touching your life.

Your lifestyle can be affected by your health. Pitta or vata doshas should find time to create a calming and restful ambience in which to relax and wind down.

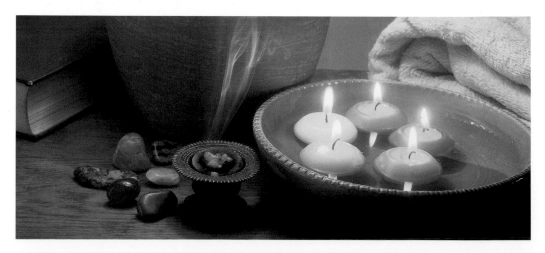

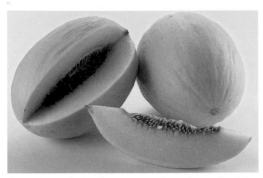

If you belong to the vata/pitta type, eat plenty of sweet, ripe fruits, such as melons and oranges, when they are in season.

Pitta/Kapha – Kapha/Pitta

This is a combination of the fire, water and earth elements. If you belong to this dual type, follow the kapha eating and living plan during the winter months and during spells of cold, damp weather, and take note of the pitta plan during the summer months, and during hot, humid weather.

You should always choose foods that are pungent and astringent, such as onions, celery, lemons, dandelion, mustard greens and watercress, and eat fresh fruit and vegetables. All fruit juices should be diluted with water or milk. Suitable teas for the pitta/kapha – kapha/pitta type include bancha twig, blackberry, dandelion, jasmine, licorice (not to be used if you suffer from high blood pressure or oedema) and spearmint. The herbs, spices and flavourings that apply to the pitta/kapha type include coriander, dill leaves, fennel, kudzu, orange peel, parsley, rosewater, and sprigs of refreshing spearmint.

Vata/Kapha – Kapha/Vata

Vata/kapha is a combination of ether, air, water and earth. You should follow the kapha eating and living plan during the winter and spring months, and during cold, damp weather. You should stick to the vata plan during the autumn and summer months, and during any cold, dry windy spells.

Since the vata/kapha type is cold, you should therefore be encouraged to have plenty of pungent, hot and spicy foods. Chinese and Eastern cuisine is a "must". Good examples of suitable foods include artichokes, asparagus, mustard greens, parsnips, summer and winter squashes and watercress. Vegetables with seeds should be well cooked with the appropriate vata spices to minimize any possible aggravation.

It is equally important to eat plenty of fresh seasonal fruits, and they include apricots, berries, cherries, lemons, mangoes, peaches and strawberries. The vata/kapha type should be very careful to avoid a mono-diet of brown rice.

The herbs and spices for this particular type include allspice, anise, asafoetida (hing), basil, black pepper, basil, cinnamon, coriander, cumin, curry powder, garlic, nutmeg, poppy seeds, saffron and vanilla.

Tridosha

In very rare instances a person may score more or less equally for all three doshas, revealing themselves to be all three types, or what is known as "tridosha" (literally, three-doshas). If you are this interesting combination of three doshas you will require a specially formulated tridoshic diet and living plan. Since your make-up is more elaborate than for single types, your plan is accordingly more interesting and varied. The onus is on you, however, to closely follow the seasonal changes and modify the agenda as appropriate, making sensible, sensitive modifications. Being a tridosha involves quite a degree of self-discipline, and a clever ability to switch promptly between all three lifestyle plans.

Always eat according to the weather and to your personal circumstances. For example, on hot days, and during the spring and summer months, follow the pitta plan; on cold days and during the winter months, follow the kapha plan; and during the late summer and autumn, or on windy days or during spells of cold dry weather, follow the vata plan.

If you find that you fall into this highly unusual, remarkable category, it will certainly be worthwhile seeking out and consulting an Ayurvedic practitioner to find out more about what being a tridosha entails.

Pitta/kapha – kapha/pitta foods include curry leaves or powder, garam masala, mint, orange peel oil and rosewater.

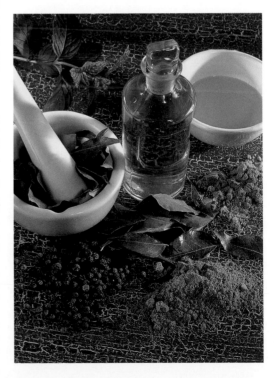

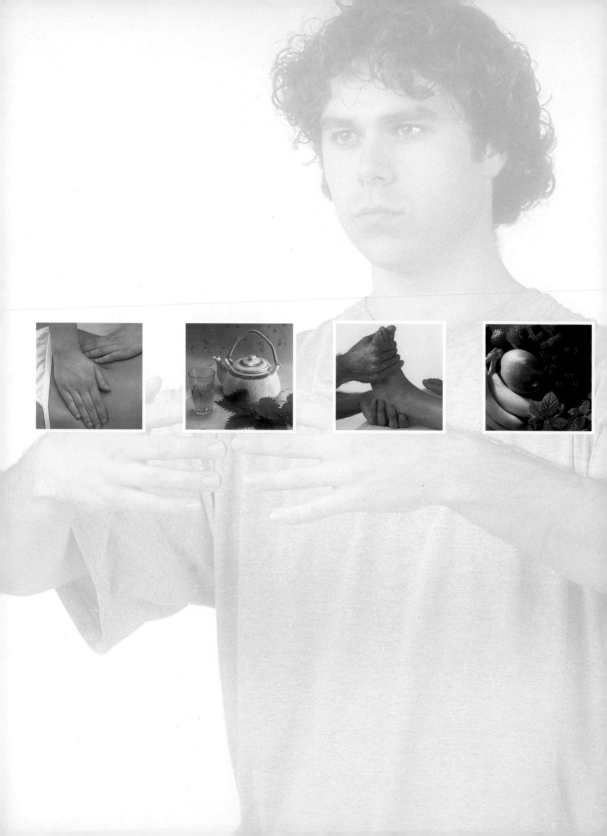

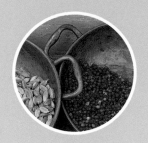

ayurvedic treatments
ayurvedic treatments

ayurvedic treatments

The entire basis and the whole concept of Ayurvedic treatment is dietary; put bluntly, diet is exactly what it all leads back to – the tried and tested use and combination of specific foods. Fortunately, several excellent, imaginative Ayurvedic cookbooks with a wide range of tasty recipes have been published, and they are definitely well worth tracking down, collecting and studying if you want to learn more about Ayurvedic nutrition. They will make a great difference at meal times.

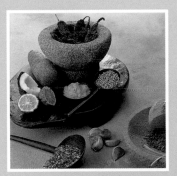

The following pages have been divided into several sections with the express purpose of outlining the basic characteristics of each type. This includes a wealth of vital information which forms the backbone, the foundation, and the essential core of the Ayurvedic approach. It deals with all kinds of related emotions, and the treatment systems closely associated with and most pertinent to each dosha. It also describes and explains the many symptoms of excess, together with a huge wealth of detail about what you should and should not be eating, which colours you really ought to be wearing, the scents and oils you should be using, the herbs and spices most beneficial to you, and the tonic recipes for each type, whether vata, pitta, or kapha.

In addition, there are key massage techniques, for example showing you how to follow the direction of the colon when massaging the stomach with brahmi oil, and which gem and crystal you should be working with in order to help you to reduce any excess levels in your dosha(s), thereby making sure they have a balanced, healthy relationship.

To the novice some of these ideas might seem slightly daunting, especially if you come from a background in which traditional forms of Western medicine have a stranglehold, but once they and the language in which they are expressed become familiar, you will see that the principles are actually very simple; they spell out some highly relevant advice. All you then have to do is to follow the right plan, whether you are trying to reduce an excess, or wish to build up and maintain the right balance in your system.

Once you become familiar with the many excellent Ayurvedic treatments, you can become slightly more adventurous. There is absolutely no reason why you should not start making up your own tonic recipes for your own body type. This is easily done by combining ingredients from the appropriate eating plan, and using recommended herbs and spices to enhance the healing.

the digestive system

One of the main cornerstones of Ayurvedic theory and medicine is that the gastro-intestinal tract (GI) is by far the most important and crucial part of the body because it is considered to be the focal point, or the principal seat, of the doshas. Vata is formed inside the colon, pitta in the small intestine, and kapha inside the stomach. In other words, this tract has extra dimensions not recognized by traditional medicine.

Constipation

Drink warm liquids; hot water is acceptable, but not chilled water. The best herbs for constipation are triphala and satisabgol (psyllium husks). (Do not use triphala if you are pregnant or suffering from ulcers of the GI.) Triphala is a combination of three herbal fruits, each of which has a rejuvenating effect in relation to one of the doshas. Satisabgol is a demulcent laxative. It is gentle and soothing and holds moisture in the colon, thus helping vata, which is known to be quite dry and cold. Use satisabgol with triphala; they complement each other well.

Gas, Bloating, Colic

These symptoms are usually related to constipation. Ideally food should pass through the system in 24 hours. If it is left for much longer the process of fermentation begins, which causes a build-up of gas. The traditional herbal remedy for this is hingvastak, a mix of asafoetida, pippali, ginger, black pepper, cumin, wild celery seeds and rock salt. Another traditional remedy is a massage with brahmi oil. It restores and relaxes the nervous system.

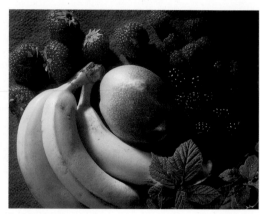

Eating a healthy vata diet can aid many vata problems associated with the gastro-intestinal tract.

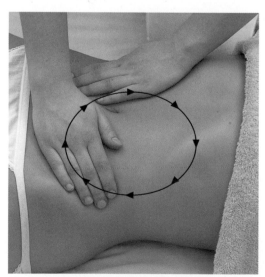

When massaging, follow the direction of the colon – from lower left, across the abdomen, up to the right and across to the left.

Acidity/Heartburn

Sip aloe vera juice (without any citric acid added). Add fresh and dried coriander (cilantro), turmeric, saffron, coconut, fennel or peppermint to your diet. Shatavari (Asparagus racemosus), licorice (not to be used with high blood pressure or oedema) and amalaki are all used in traditional Ayurveda medicine in order to balance unwelcome levels of acidity.

Diarrhoea

Pitta diarrhoea is generally hot, and often yellowish and foul-smelling. Diarrhoea is mainly related to pitta but can sometimes be caused by other factors, such as high toxicity (ama), stress or emotional factors. Persistent symptoms must always be dealt with by an experienced, professional physician. If you have diarrhoea, avoid eating hot spices and carefully follow the pitta plan. Eat abstemiously if at all, drinking plenty of fluids. A simple straightforward diet of rice, split mung dhal and vegetables is most suitable for the pitta dosha, taken while symptoms last.

Persistent Hunger/Increased Appetite

In general, follow the pitta plan as outlined and use aloe vera juice as above. Increase relaxation, meditation and yoga. Also, have a long massage with brahmi oil. If strong symptoms persist, do please promptly consult your physician.

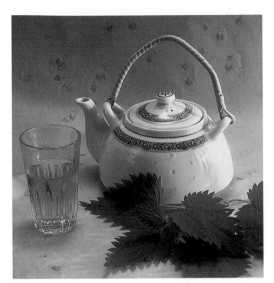

Nettle tea is very good at balancing the digestive system and can help to alleviate pitta conditions such as diarrhoea.

Nausea

Nausea can quite simply be defined as the strong sensation of needing to vomit. It might not actually result in vomiting, but produces a queasy, lingering feeling that needs to be quickly relieved. It certainly is not pleasant.

Ginger and cardamom tea is often very good at calming nausea. To make it, peel and thinly slice a piece of fresh ginger, add five cardamom pods and pour boiled spring water over them. Leave to stand for about five minutes, and then stir and drink while still refreshing and hot.

Ginger is also what is known as a carminative and a stimulant. This means that it has two key abilities, first to combat any intestinal bloating, and second to speed up processes in the GI so that balance is soon restored.

During the winter and spring seasons when kapha is seasonally high, dried ginger can be blended with some boiled spring water and a little fresh honey to help keep the digestive system active and moving. This also has the excellent effect of helping to reduce the possible risk of colds, coughs and flu, and any other winter bugs that might otherwise keep you confined to the bed or house for a number of days.

Cardamom (common in southern India as well as other tropical areas, and now freely available in supermarkets) can be used for kapha and vata digestive conditions. However, it can only be used in small amounts because it can quickly aggravate pitta, or bring about a high level of pitta excess.

As with all the recommended foods, herbs and spices, the purer the quality, the more beneficial they will be. Therefore, try to buy top quality, fresh organic herbs and spices whenever it is possible. You will immediately appreciate the difference.

The Doshas and the Gastro-intestinal Tract

Kapha

Typical kapha conditions of the GI include poor appetite – kapha tends to be low in agni (digestive fire), which can create a slow metabolism and weight gain; nausea; a build-up of mucus, leading to colds, sinus problems, coughs and flu; and poor circulation, resulting in a build-up of toxicity (ama). Follow the kapha plan and eat plenty of hot spices, such as chilli peppers, garlic, ginger and black pepper, until the condition clears, after which you should reduce your intake of hot spices. Herbs for kapha conditions of the GI include trikatu ("three hot things"), to be taken or added to meals. This contains pippali, ginger and black pepper. You should also have plenty of vigorous exercise.

Vata

Regular daily bowel movements are a sign of a healthy GI. Typical vata conditions of the GI include constipation, gas/flatulence, and tension – cramps or spasms, such as irritable bowel syndrome.

Pitta

Pitta digestion tends to be fast and "burns" food. This is made worse by anger or frustration. Begin a pitta-reducing diet and eat in a calm and relaxed way. Typical pitta conditions of the gastro-intestinal tract include acidity and heartburn, symptomized by belching and acid indigestion; diarrhoea or frequent loose bowel movements, and constant hunger, accompanied by consequent irritability.

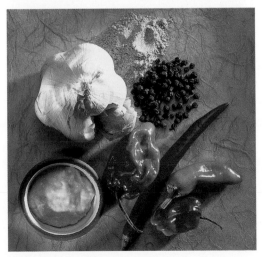

Hot kapha dietary spices.

common problems
It is quite clear that the forms taken by various commonly occurring illnesses, and the appropriate remedies, will vary according to whether you have a vata, pitta or kapha dosha. The following sections therefore aim to give you individually a plan of action, setting out all the do's and do not's. Note that in the case of any persistent, or indeed serious illness, you must immediately contact a qualified professional expert.

Insomnia
Any vata-increasing influence can contribute to your insomnia, including regular travel, stress, an irregular lifestyle, and the excessive use of stimulants such as tea and coffee. The herbs used to treat vata-based insomnia are brahmi (Centella), jatamansi, ashwagandha (Withania somnifera) and nutmeg. Any good massage using brahmi oil will also produce considerable, quickly noticed benefits.

Insomnia in the pitta dosha is brought on by anger, jealousy, frustration, fever, excess sun or heat. Follow the pitta plan, which is cooling, and take brahmi, jatamansi, bhringaraj (Eclipta alba), shatavari and aloe vera juice. Massage brahmi oil into the head and feet. Again, this is marvellously refreshing.

As kapha types like to sleep and tend to be rather sleepy and sluggish, they rarely suffer from attacks of insomnia.

Headache/Migraine
Vata headaches cause extreme pain and are related to anxiety and tension. Relevant treatments include triphala to clear any congestion, jatamansi, brahmi and calamus.

Pitta headaches are associated with heat or burning sensations, flushed skin and a visual sensitivity to light. They are related to anger, frustration or irritability, and will be connected to the liver and gall bladder. Treatments are brahmi, turmeric and aloe vera juice. Kapha headaches are dull and heavy and can cause nausea. There may also be congestion, such as catarrh. Have a stimulating massage with minimal oil.

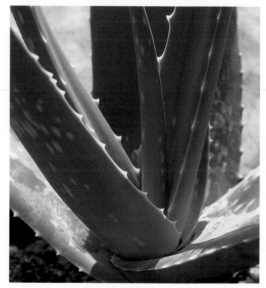

Juice from aloe vera plants can be used to combat sleeplessness.

Colds
A tendency to mucus production or catarrh/phlegm is unpleasant for the sufferer, and is usually the result of poor digestion of foods in the stomach which increases ama (toxicity) and kapha. In general, kapha is generally considered the most highly effective dosha.

Vata-type colds involve dry symptoms, such as a dry cough or dry throat. Herbs for vata coughs and colds are ginger, cumin, pippali, tulsi (holy basil, Ocimum sanctum), cloves and peppermint, licorice (not to be used with high blood pressure or oedema), shatavari and ashwagandha. Put one or two drops of sesame oil up each nostril, and then follow the vata plan until all the symptoms are seen to subside.

Pitta-type colds involve more heat, the face is usually red and there may even be a fever. The mucus is often yellow and can actually contain traces of blood. Herbs for tackling pitta coughs and colds include peppermint and various other mints, sandalwood, chrysanthemum and small quantities of tulsi (holy basil). Follow the pitta plan until your symptoms begin to subside.

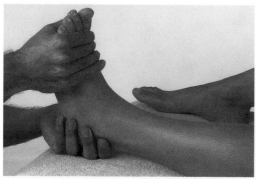

A foot massage with brahmi oil will often relieve insomnia.

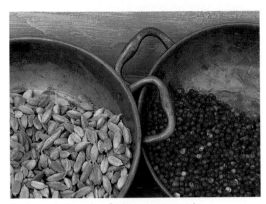

Cardamom pods are beneficial to vata-type coughs.

Kapha colds are thick and mucusy, with a feeling of heaviness in the head and/or body. Avoid cold, damp weather and exposure to cold and damp conditions. Eliminate sugar, refined foods, meat and nuts, dairy products, bread, fats and oils from the diet and use plenty of hot spices. Drink a spiced tea of hot lemon, ginger and cinnamon with cloves or tulsi, sweetened with a little raw honey. Herbs for kapha colds are ginger, cinnamon, pippali, tulsi (holy basil), cloves and peppermint. Saunas and hot baths will help to increase the heat of the kapha person, but they should not be used in excess as this would actually increase the pitta too much. Follow the kapha plan until the symptoms subside.

Coughs

Vata coughs are dry and irritated with very little mucus, the chief symptom being a painful cough often accompanied by a dry mouth. Herbs and spices for the vata cough include licorice (do not use this if you have high blood pressure or oedema), shatavari, ashwagandha and cardamom. Follow the vata plan until the symptoms subside.

Pitta coughs are usually associated with a lot of phlegm. The chest is congested and very uncomfortable, but the mucus cannot be brought up properly. There is often fever or heat, combined with a burning sensation in the chest or throat. High fevers should be treated by a physician, and people suffering with asthma should consult their doctor immediately if a cough or cold leads to wheezing and difficult breathing. The best herbs for pitta coughs include peppermint, tulsi (holy basil) and sandalwood. Follow the pitta plan until the symptoms have completely subsided.

With kapha coughs, the patient usually brings up lots of phlegm, and suffers a loss of appetite combined with nausea. The chest is loaded with mucus, but this may not be coughed up because the kapha individual is likely to feel tired. Treatments for kapha coughs are raw honey, lemon, cloves and chyawanprash (a herbal jam). Follow the kapha plan until the symptoms subside, increasing your intake of hot spices, and do try to use trikatu powder. Also keep warm.

Skin Problems

These are often caused by internal conditions of toxicity (ama) and are mainly related to the pitta dosha. Vata skin problems will be dry and rough. Avoid letting the skin dry out. Herbal remedies for vata skin are triphala and satisabgol. Pitta skin problems will be red and swollen, often with a yellow head. Avoid sun, heat or hot baths, and increase your intake of salads. Follow the pitta plan and add turmeric, coriander and saffron to your diet. The remedies are manjishta (Rubia cordifolia), kutki (Picrohiza kurroa), turmeric and aloe vera juice. Kapha skin problems involve blood congestion which can cause the skin to form thick and mucusy whiteheads. Increase your level of exercise, and follow the kapha plan. Treatments should always include a small amount of calamus with some dry ginger and quantities of turmeric.

Urinary Infections

Excess cold water, tea, coffee, and alcoholic drinks will weaken the kidneys. Salt, sugar or foods that are rich in calcium, such as dairy products or spinach, will similarly tend to weaken and toxify the kidneys. The best kidney tonic to use in Ayurveda is shilajit, a mineral-rich compound from the Himalayan mountains, but avoid it if you suffer from kidney stones. Pregnant women, children or those on medication should consult an Ayurvedic practitioner before treatment.

Cystitis

In vata people, cystitis will tend to be less intense. Remedies are shilajit (to be avoided if you suffer from kidney stones) with bala (Sida cordifolia), ashwagandha and shatavari.

Cystitis is mainly a pitta condition because it burns and is hot. Follow the pitta plan, using plenty of coriander (cilantro) and avoiding hot spices. Remedies include aloe vera juice (not to be used in pregnancy), lime juice, coconut and sandalwood. Kapha-type cystitis is accompanied by congestion and mucus in the urinary tract. The treatments are cinnamon, trikatu combined with shilajit, gokshura and gokshurdi guggul.

It is worth having a supply of fresh mint and other herbs to hand for many of the common Ayurvedic treatments.

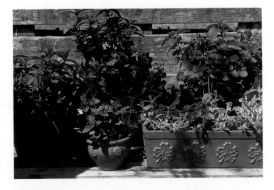

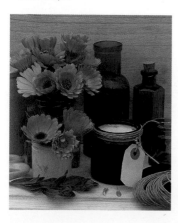

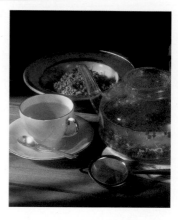

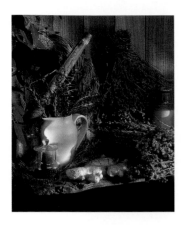
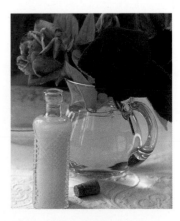

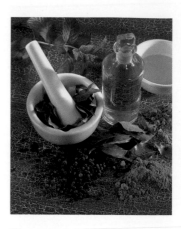

Picture credits

*The publishers would particularly like to thank the
following photographers for the use of their pictures:*
Michelle Garrett, Alistair Hughes, Lucy Mason and
Debbie Patterson.

*Thanks also to the following libraries for supplying
pictures:* A-Z Botanical Collection Ltd: 35BL; 47TR;
52BL; 60BL; 61BL, BR; 62BR; 63TL; 65TM. Bruce
Coleman Collection: 62BM; 63TM; 64BM. Frank
Lane Photographic Agency: 39BM. Garden &
Wildlife Matters: 38TL; 59BM. The Garden Picture
Library: 36BL, TR; 38TM; 39BR; 63BL. Images
Colour Library: 74B. Harry Smith Collection:
53BL; 61TM; 64TL, TR; 65BM. Tony Stone Images:
35BR; 68T, B ,71B; 72B; 78B; 82B.

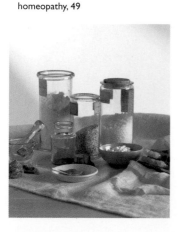

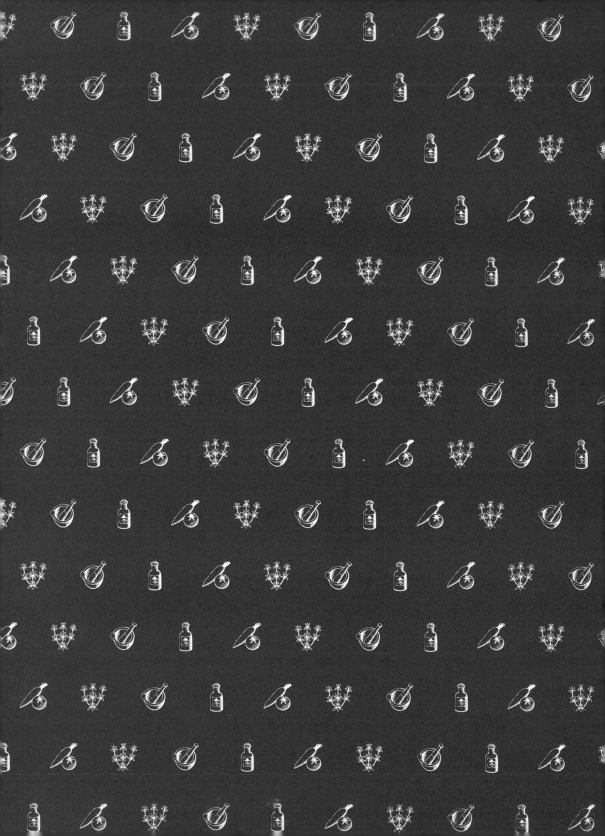

How Science Works

Ideas

Sometimes our opinions are based on our own prejudices; what we personally like or dislike.

At other times, our opinions can be based on scientific evidence. Reliable and valid evidence can be used to back up our own opinions.

Variables

- An **independent** variable is the variable that we choose to change to see what happens.
- A **dependent** variable is the variable that we measure.
- A **continuous** variable (e.g. time or mass) can have any numerical value.
- An **ordered** variable (e.g. small, medium, large) can be listed in order.
- A **discrete** variable can have any value that is a whole number, e.g. 1, 2.
- A **categoric** variable is a variable that can be labelled, e.g. red, blue.
- We use **line graphs** to present data where the independent variable and the dependent variable are both continuous. A line of best fit can be used to show the relationship between variables.
- **Bar graphs** are used to present data when the independent variable is categoric and the dependent variable is continuous.

Evidence

Evidence should be:

- **reliable and repeatable** (if you do it again you get the same result)
- **accurate** (close to the true value).

Scientists often try to find links between variables.

Links can be:

- causal (a change in one variable produces a change in the other variable)
- a chance occurrence
- due to an association, where both of the observed variables are linked by a third variable.

We can use our existing models and ideas to suggest why something happens. This is called a **hypothesis**. We can use this hypothesis to make a **prediction** that can be tested.

When data is collected, if it does not back up our original models and ideas, we need to check that the data is valid. If it is valid, we need to go back and change our original models and ideas.

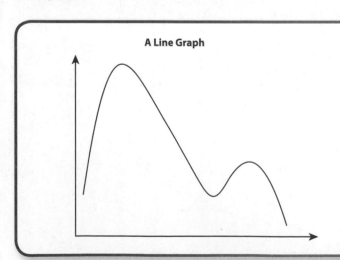

A Line Graph

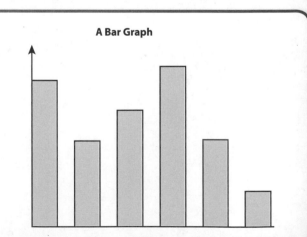

A Bar Graph

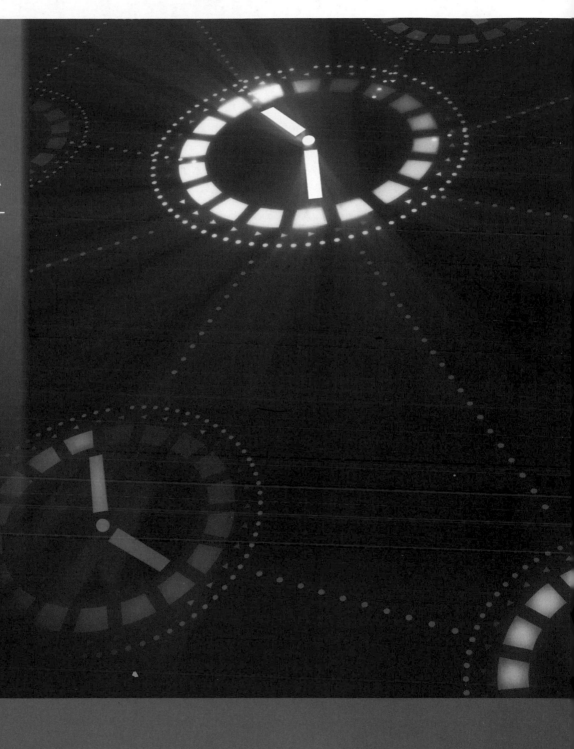

GCSE
IN A
WEEK

Physics

Caroline Reynolds and Dan Foulder

Revision Planner

Science in Society

Sometimes scientists investigate subjects that have social consequences, e.g. food safety. When this happens, decisions may be based on a combination of the evidence and other factors, such as bias or political considerations.

Although science is helping us to understand more about our world, there are still some questions that we cannot answer, such as 'Is there life on other planets?'. Some questions are for everyone in society, not just scientists, to answer, such as 'Should we clone humans?'.

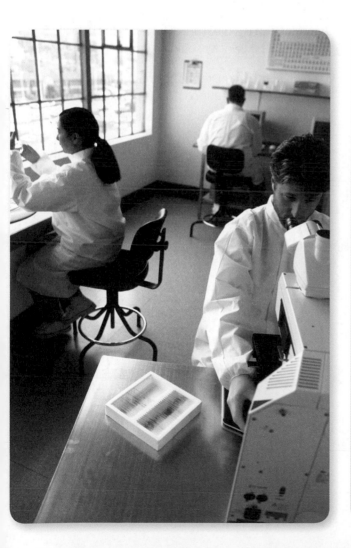

SUMMARY

- Scientists carry out experiments with a range of different types of variables.
- Scientific evidence should be reliable and repeatable, and accurate.
- Links between variables can be causal (due to another variable) or just occur by chance.
- Scientists use hypotheses to make predictions that can be tested.

QUESTIONS

QUICK TEST

1. What is an independent variable?

2. What is a dependent variable?

3. What is an ordered variable?

4. What is a discrete variable?

5. What does accurate mean?

EXAM PRACTICE

1. A student carries out an experiment to find out how the force applied to a spring affects the length of the spring.

   a) What is the independent variable? **(1 mark)**

   b) What is the dependent variable? **(1 mark)**

   c) Suggest a variable that must be controlled to make it a fair test. **(1 mark)**

Motion

Speed

Speed is a measure of how fast something is going; it is usually measured in m/s. For example, an object that covers a distance of 3 m every second has a speed of 3 m/s.

$$\text{Speed} = \frac{\text{distance}}{\text{time}}$$

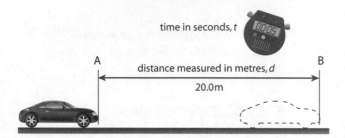

time in seconds, t

A

distance measured in metres, d

20.0 m

B

If the car above travels a distance AB of 20.0 m in a time t of 5.0 s, its average speed is:

$$\frac{20.0\,\text{m}}{5.0\,\text{s}} = 4.0\,\text{m/s}$$

Speed cameras generally take two photographs a certain time apart and near marked lines on a road. This is because they need to measure the distance travelled in a certain time.

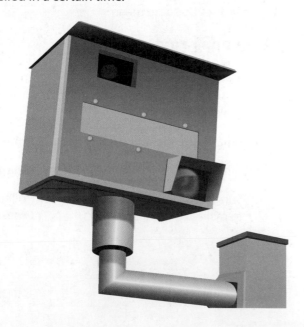

Velocity

Velocity is a measure of how fast something is going in a given direction. Its units are also m/s. The difference between speed and velocity is that velocity includes the direction, whereas speed does not.

$$\text{Average velocity} = \frac{\text{displacement}}{\text{time}}$$

Speed has magnitude (size) only; it is a **scalar quantity**.

Velocity has magnitude **and** direction; it is a **vector quantity**.

Acceleration

Acceleration is a measure of how fast the velocity is changing. The velocity could be increasing or decreasing.

- If velocity is constant, the change in velocity is zero and the acceleration is 0 m/s per second or 0 m/s^2.
- If velocity increases by 1 m/s every second, the acceleration is 1 m/s^2.
- If velocity decreases by 2 m/s every second, the acceleration is –2 m/s^2; this is called deceleration.

Acceleration is calculated using the following equation:

$$\text{Acceleration} = \frac{\text{change in velocity}}{\text{time taken}}$$

$$or \quad a = \frac{(v - u)}{t}$$

where v = final velocity and u = initial velocity

To measure acceleration, the velocity must be measured at two different times. This can be done with light gates.

The data processor measures the velocity at two different points and measures the time between them.

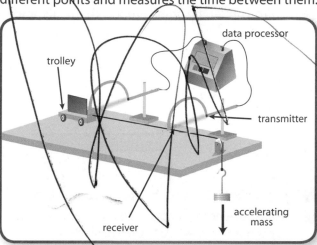

The data processor calculates the acceleration using the equation:

$$a = \frac{(v - u)}{t}$$

Example

A cart starts at the first laser. The cart is at rest so its speed is 0 m/s. It's then pushed and passed through a second laser five seconds later. The data processor gave the final speed of the cart as 2.0 m/s. Calculate the acceleration of the cart.

$$\text{Acceleration} = \frac{(5 - 0)}{5}$$

$$= \textbf{1 m/s}^2$$

Sometimes, only the direction of a moving body changes. For example, if a planet rotates around the Sun at a constant speed:

● the speed is constant
● the velocity is changing because the direction is changing
● the planet is accelerating because the velocity is changing.

SUMMARY

● $\text{Speed} = \frac{\text{distance}}{\text{time}}$
● $\text{Average velocity} = \frac{\text{displacement}}{\text{time}}$
● Speed is a scalar quantity; velocity is a vector quantity as it has a direction.
● $\text{Acceleration} = \frac{\text{change in velocity}}{\text{time taken}}$

QUESTIONS

QUICK TEST

1. Why do speed cameras generally take two photographs a certain time apart and near marked lines on a road?

2. What is the equation that relates average velocity, displacement and time?

3. Find the average velocity of a car that travels 300 m in 15 s.

4. What is the difference between speed and velocity?

5. When a car turns a corner at constant speed, is there a change in velocity?

EXAM PRACTICE

1. **a)** What is the acceleration of a car that accelerates from 10 m/s to 30 m/s in 4.0 s?
   (1 mark)

   b) Find the deceleration of the car if it slows down from 30 m/s to 0 m/s in 3.0 s. **(1 mark)**

2. Two trains set off from the same point. One had a negative velocity compared to the other. What does this show? **(1 mark)**

3. If a data processor is used to measure the acceleration of a vehicle, what **three** pieces of information does it need? **(3 marks)**

Graphs for Motion

Distance–Time Graphs

Distance–time graphs show how the distance from a start point changes over time.

The graph below shows the distance a car travels from a start point over a period of ten seconds.

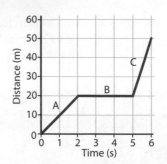

A: The car is moving away from its start point at a constant speed, so the distance increases over time. The car's speed is equal to the gradient of the graph. The car moves 20 m in 2 s, so the gradient can be found by $\frac{20\,m}{2\,s} = 10\,m/s$. The car's speed is 10 m/s.

B: The car is stationary. It is a constant distance from the start point, so the line on the graph is flat.

C: The car sets off again moving away from its start point. The car is moving faster than it was from 0–2 seconds, so the line is steeper. The gradient this time is $\frac{30\,m}{1\,s} = 30\,m/s$.

The rocket shown by the graph below is accelerating. This means its speed is increasing over time. This is shown on a distance–time graph by an increasing gradient.

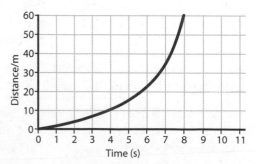

Velocity–Time Graphs

A **velocity–time graph** shows how the speed or velocity of an object changes with time.

● The **gradient** is equal to the **acceleration**.
● The **area** under the graph is equal to the **distance** travelled.

This velocity–time graph is for a car. It shows a steady speed of 5.0 m/s.

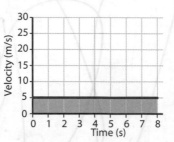

● The gradient is zero, so the acceleration is $0\,m/s^2$.
● The area under the graph is $5.0\,m/s \times 8.0\,s = 40\,m$. The car has travelled a distance of 40 m.

This graph shows more complicated motion.

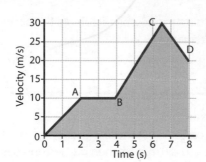

From the origin to A:

● the acceleration $= \frac{10\,m/s}{2\,s} = 5\,m/s^2$
● the distance travelled $= \frac{(10\,m/s \times 2\,s)}{2} = 10\,m$

From A to B:

● the acceleration is zero
● the distance travelled is $(10\,m/s \times 2\,s) = 20\,m$

From B to C:

● the acceleration is $\frac{20\,m/s}{2.5\,s} = 8\,m/s^2$
● the distance is $(10\,m/s \times 2.5\,s) + (\frac{(20\,m/s \times 2.5\,s)}{2}) = 50\,m$

From C to D the gradient is negative, so the acceleration is negative. The car is slowing down, or decelerating. The total distance travelled is 80 m.

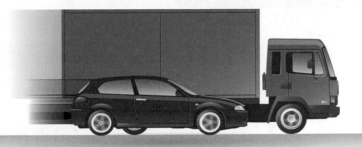

SUMMARY

● On a distance–time graph:

 – a flat line indicates the object is stationary

 – the steeper the line, the faster the object is moving.

● On a velocity–time graph:

 – the gradient is equal to the acceleration

 – the area under the graph is equal to the distance travelled.

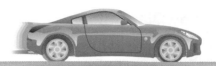

QUESTIONS

QUICK TEST

1. The graph opposite shows a motorbike travelling around a circuit.

   a) At what point on the graph is:

   i) the motorbike stationary?

   ii) the motorbike moving away from the start point at a constant speed?

   iii) the motorbike returning to the start point at a constant speed?

   b) Calculate the speed the motorbike is travelling between A–B.

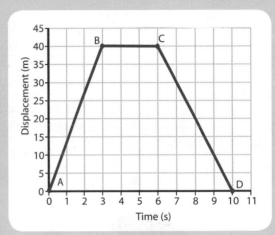

EXAM PRACTICE

1. The graph opposite shows the velocity of a car over time. Calculate:

   a) the car's deceleration from D–E.   **(1 mark)**

   b) how far the car travelled from A–C.   **(2 marks)**

   c) the maximum acceleration during the 10 seconds shown.   **(2 marks)**

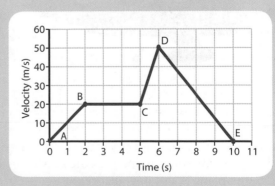

When Forces Combine

Free Body Diagrams

This **free body diagram** shows the forces acting on a girl standing on a plank. There are other forces acting on the plank and on the ground, but the free body diagram only considers the forces that act on a single body (in this case, the girl).

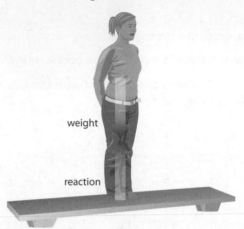

The girl experiences the force due to gravity acting downwards and the reaction force of the plank acting upwards. These forces are the same size, so they cancel out. There is no net force and the girl stays still. The girl is in **equilibrium**.

The picture below shows a free body diagram for a plane at constant velocity.

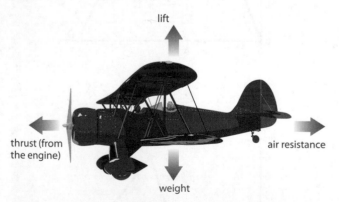

The upward and downward forces on the plane cancel out. The forwards and backwards forces also cancel out. Because the plane is already moving, this means that the plane continues to move at the same constant velocity. The plane is also in equilibrium.

The picture below shows a free body diagram for a skydiver.

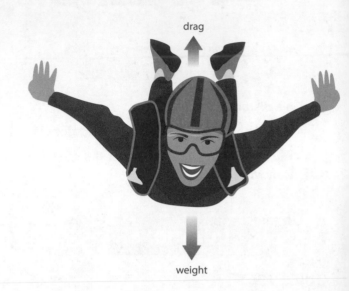

The skydiver experiences weight and **air resistance** (or drag). When these forces are not equal, i.e. weight is more than drag, there is a net **resultant force** downwards.

For example, if weight equals 400 N and the air resistance equals 80 N, the net or resultant force is 320 N in a downward direction. The skydiver is accelerating downwards. He is not in equilibrium.

Note that these two forces are in opposite directions. Therefore, the resultant force is found by subtraction. If the forces are in the same direction, the resultant force is found by adding.

Action and Reaction

Whenever two bodies interact, the forces they exert on each other are equal and opposite.

An **action force** produces an equal and opposite **reaction force**. These forces are always:

- equal in magnitude
- opposite in direction
- the same type of force
- on different bodies.

SUMMARY

- To calculate a resultant force from two separate forces:
    - If the forces are acting in the same direction, add them together.
    - If the forces are acting in opposite directions, subtract one from the other.
- An action force produces an equal and opposite reaction force.

QUESTIONS

QUICK TEST

1. What is a free body diagram?

2. **a)** Sketch a free body diagram for a skydiver accelerating.

   b) If the weight in your diagram is equal to 550 N and the air resistance is equal to 150 N, what is the resultant force on the skydiver?

3. **a)** Consider the man opposite. Why does the boat move backwards as he steps forwards?

   b) Identify the action and the reaction forces for the man and the boat.

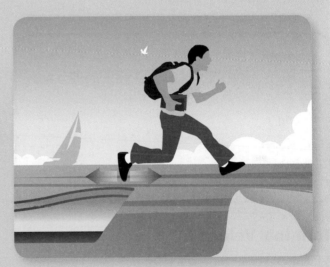

EXAM PRACTICE

1. The diagram opposite shows the forces acting on a cyclist as he cycles down the road.

   a) What is the name of the force that is acting against the cyclist's forward motion? **(1 mark)**

   b) Calculate the resultant force. **(1 mark)**

   c) Explain what would happen to the cyclist if both forces were equal. **(2 marks)**

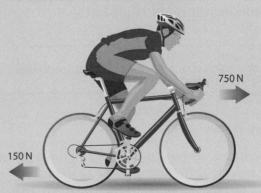

750 N

150 N

Forces and Motion

Resultant Force

If the **resultant force** on a body is zero, it will remain stationary or continue to move at the same speed in the same direction.

If the resultant force on a body is not zero, it will accelerate in the direction of the resultant force.

Acceleration is always caused by a resultant force.

The acceleration can be calculated as follows:

> Force = mass × acceleration $F = ma$

The units of force are Newtons (N).

> **Example**
> A 2 kg toy car is pushed so it accelerates at 0.5 m/s^2. What is the force acting on it?
>
> $F = ma$
>
> $F = 2 \times 0.5$
>
> $F = \mathbf{1\ N}$

Terminal Velocity

A falling skydiver experiences a force called weight that acts towards the centre of the Earth.

> Weight = mass × gravitational field strength (g)

On Earth, g is about 10 N/kg.

Initially, weight is the only force acting on the skydiver. As the skydiver falls, **friction** with the air particles increases. This is called **air resistance** (or drag). This opposes the force due to gravity.

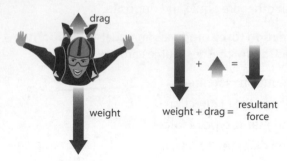

These two forces combine to produce a resultant force in a downward direction. The skydiver accelerates.

The acceleration produces increased velocity. This produces more drag.

The acceleration continues to increase velocity and hence drag. Eventually, drag becomes equal in magnitude to weight.

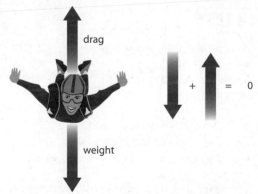

Now the skydiver has reached **terminal velocity**, which is the maximum velocity attainable. The skydiver continues to fall with constant velocity; there is no further acceleration. The forces are balanced, the skydiver is in equilibrium and the resultant force is zero.

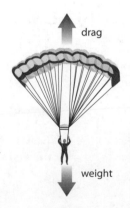

An object with greater surface area or a less streamlined shape has greater drag. When the skydiver opens their parachute, the force of drag on them increases. This causes them to decelerate to a much lower constant terminal velocity.

The graph below shows how the velocity of a skydiver changes as they fall.

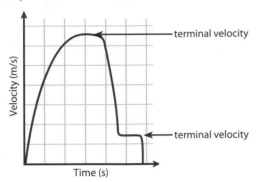

The skydiver accelerates as they fall until they reach a maximum velocity (terminal velocity). They then open their parachute. This causes a large increase in drag, which causes a large deceleration before they reach a new, much lower, terminal velocity. They then land so their velocity is zero.

When there is no atmosphere, such as in space, there is no air resistance.

Forces for Circular Motion

An object moving in a circle is accelerating due to its direction changing.

The resultant force that causes this acceleration acts towards the centre of the circle. For a mass on a string, this force is provided by the tension in the string. For an orbiting planet, this force is provided by the gravitational pull on the planet.

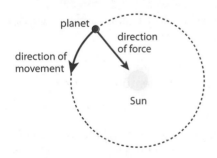

The **centripetal force** needed to make a body perform circular motion increases as:

- the mass of the body increases
- the speed of the body increases
- the radius of the circle decreases.

SUMMARY

- **Force = mass × acceleration**
- **Weight = mass × gravitational field strength**
- **When the drag of a falling object equals its weight, it is at terminal velocity. This means it will continue to fall at a constant velocity.**
- **Drag is affected by how streamlined an object is.**
- **The centripetal force of an object is dependent on the mass of the object, the speed of the object and the size of its orbit.**

QUESTIONS

QUICK TEST

1. A 20 N force is applied to an object of 2.0 kg. What is the acceleration?

2. What is the direction of the force needed for circular motion?

3. Name **three** ways of increasing the centripetal force required to make a body perform circular motion.

EXAM PRACTICE

1. What is the weight on Earth of an object with a mass of 9 kg? **(1 mark)**

2. A warehouse worker pushes a crate with a mass of 30 kg along the floor with a force of 60 N. What is its initial acceleration? **(2 marks)**

3. Explain, in terms of forces, why a skydiver jumping from a plane is able to land safely.

   The quality of written communication will be assessed in your answer to this question.
   (6 marks)

Momentum and Stopping

Momentum

A faster-moving body has more kinetic energy; it also has more **momentum**.

When calculating what happens to bodies as a result of explosions or collisions, it is often more useful to think in terms of momentum than energy.

> Momentum (kgm/s) = mass (kg) × velocity (m/s)

A car of mass 1000 kg travelling at 6 m/s has momentum of 6000 kgm/s.

Momentum has **magnitude** and **direction** (it's a vector).

- When a resultant force acts on a body that is moving, or able to move, a change in momentum occurs.
- Momentum is conserved in any collision / explosion, providing no external forces act on the bodies.

Example
A trolley of 1.0 kg travelling at 3.0 m/s collides with a stationary trolley of mass 2.0 kg. If, after the collision, the first trolley stops and the second trolley begins to move, find the velocity of the second trolley.

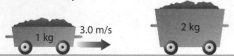

> Momentum before = Momentum afterwards

$(1.0 \, \text{kg} \times 3.0 \, \text{m/s}) + (2.0 \, \text{kg} \times 0 \, \text{m/s}) =$
$(1.0 \, \text{kg} \times 0 \, \text{m/s}) + (2.0 \, \text{kg} \times \text{speed after})$

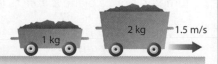

Velocity of second trolley after collision = **1.5 m/s**

Momentum is conserved when a rocket is propelled through space. The momentum of fuel ejected in a certain time is equal to the change in momentum of the rocket during that time. Momentum is also conserved in collisions in sport, for example when a racket hits a tennis ball.

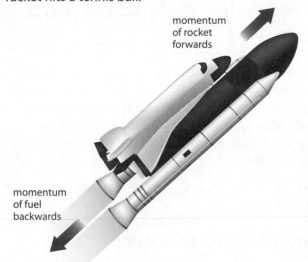

momentum of rocket forwards

momentum of fuel backwards

Stopping

- A vehicle at greater speed requires more braking force to stop in a certain distance.
- A vehicle of greater mass requires more braking force to stop in a certain distance.

The force needed to stop a car is found by considering the change in momentum:

> Change in momentum = force × time

For a car of mass 1200 kg travelling at 20 m/s to stop, the momentum change is 1200 kg × 20 m/s = 24 000 kgm/s.

To stop in 6 s the brakes must exert a force of:

$$\frac{24\,000 \, \text{kgm/s}}{6 \, \text{s}} = 4000 \, \text{N}$$

If the braking time is reduced to 3 s, the force is doubled to 8000 N.

If the car is stopped more quickly, for example by hitting a tree, the stopping time is reduced and the force is increased further.

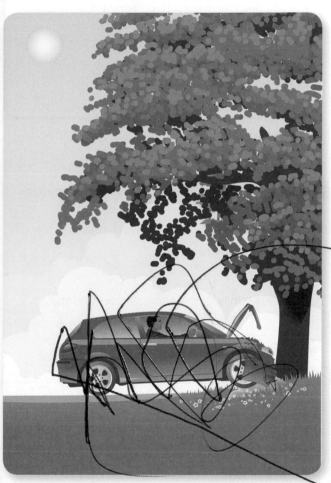

Car manufacturers use technology to increase stopping time (and stopping distance) in order to reduce the force on the passengers. Some of the features used are:

- air bags that inflate, which stop passengers more gently
- seat belts, which stop passengers hitting hard surfaces inside cars
- crumple zones that collapse steadily in a collision, which spreads the stopping over a longer time.

When stopping time (and stopping distance) is increased, deceleration is reduced. Injuries are reduced by devices changing shape and absorbing energy.

QUESTIONS

QUICK TEST

1. Find the momentum of a bicycle and rider of 75 kg travelling at 10 m/s.

2. How does force affect momentum?

3. What is a crumple zone?

EXAM PRACTICE

1. a) A trolley of mass 2.0 kg moves with a velocity of 3.0 m/s.
      Find its momentum.   **(1 mark)**

   b) The trolley collides with a stationary trolley of 1.0 kg. The trolleys stick together.
      Find their combined mass.   **(1 mark)**

   c) Calculate the total momentum of the two trolleys.   **(1 mark)**

   d) Calculate the velocity of the trolleys after the collision.   **(2 marks)**

Safe Driving

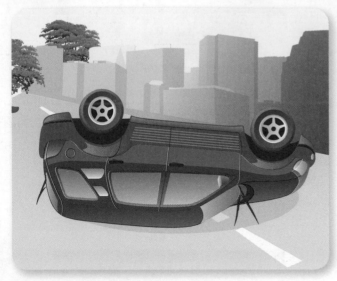

Stopping Distance

The total **stopping distance** of a car is made up of the **thinking distance** and the **braking distance**.

- Thinking distance = distance travelled between the need for braking occurring and the brakes being applied.
- Braking distance = distance taken to stop once the brakes have been applied.

> Stopping distance = thinking distance + braking distance

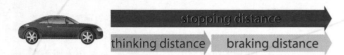

Thinking Distance

The thinking distance depends on the driver's **reaction time**, which can be affected by:

- driver tiredness
- the influence of alcohol or other drugs
- distractions or lack of concentration.

A greater speed means that a greater distance will be covered in the same time.

Example

A car is travelling at a speed of 20 m/s and the driver's reaction time is 0.4 s. What is the thinking distance?

$$\text{Distance} = \text{speed} \times \text{time}$$
$$= 20 \text{ m/s} \times 0.4 \text{ s}$$
$$= \mathbf{8.0 \text{ m}}$$

Braking Distance

The **braking distance** can be affected by:

- road conditions – **friction** is affected when roads are wet or icy
- car conditions – worn tyres, worn brakes
- the mass of the car
- speed.

Safe drivers consider the above factors and the implications on:

- the distance they are from the car in front
- speed limits.

Active and Passive Safety

Active controls make driving safer, prevent crashes from occurring, and better protect occupants during a crash.

Some active safety features are listed below:

- To stop quickly, a car needs a high braking force. This relies on the friction between the tyres and the road. If brakes are applied too hard the wheels will lock (stop turning) and the car will begin to skid. **ABS braking systems** detect this locking and automatically adjust the braking force to prevent skidding.
- **Traction control** prevents spinning of wheels when excessive acceleration or steering is applied, usually by reducing speed automatically.
- **Safety cages**.

Passive safety features reduce distractions that could lead to an accident occurring.

Some typical passive safety features include:

- electric windows
- cruise control
- paddle shift controls on the steering wheel for changing gears or the stereo
- adjustable seating.

Fuel for Cars

The main fuels used in road transport are fossil fuels such as petrol and diesel.

Electricity can be used for battery-driven cars and solar cars. These do not pollute at point of use, but the battery needs recharging, which uses electricity supplied from power stations.

Fuel consumption depends on:

- speed
- friction
- driving style
- road conditions.

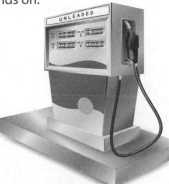

SUMMARY

- **Stopping distance is made up of thinking and braking distance.**
- **The thinking distance depends on the driver's reaction time.**
- **The braking distance depends on how quickly the brakes stop the car.**
- **Car safety measures can be active or passive.**

QUESTIONS

QUICK TEST

1. Define thinking distance.

2. Define braking distance.

3. State **two** factors that affect thinking distance.

4. What is ABS?

5. Name **three** passive safety features in a car.

EXAM PRACTICE

1. The arrow below shows the thinking and braking distance of a car.

   | Thinking distance = 12 m | Braking distance = 15 m |

   Calculate the stopping distance of the car.
   (1 mark)

2. Laura was investigating the stopping distance of cars. The variables she decided to consider were:

   - driver concentration
   - driver alcohol intake
   - mass of the car
   - condition of the car's tyres

   a) Which of the above factors affect braking distance and which affect thinking distance? **(2 marks)**

   b) Why is driver concentration a difficult variable to investigate? **(2 marks)**

3. Explain what factors would need to be considered when designing an experiment to investigate a car's fuel consumption.

   The quality of written communication will be assessed in your answer to this question.
   (6 marks)

Energy and Work

Transfer of Energy

The scientific meaning of **work** is the **transfer of energy** from one form to another or from one place to another. A light bulb does work as it changes electrical energy into heat and light. An oven does work as it transfers heat to the food. Therefore, energy is needed to do work.

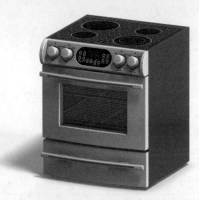

The **law of conservation of energy** states that energy can change from one form to another, but it cannot be created or destroyed.

Both energy and work are measured in **joules** (J).

In this topic, we will consider **kinetic energy** (KE) and **gravitational potential energy** (PE).

Kinetic Energy

Kinetic energy is found using the following equation:

$$\text{Kinetic energy} = \frac{1}{2} \times \text{mass} \times \text{velocity}^2$$

$$KE = \frac{1}{2} mv^2$$

All moving objects have kinetic energy. Kinetic energy is greater for objects with:

● greater speed
● greater mass.

Doubling the mass doubles the kinetic energy.

Doubling the speed quadruples the kinetic energy. This means that a car with double the speed needs about four times the braking distance.

Gravitational Potential Energy

Gravitational potential energy is found using the following equation:

$$\text{Gravitational potential energy transferred} = \text{mass} \times \text{gravitational field strength} \times \text{change in height}$$

$$PE = mgh$$

Gravitational potential energy is greater for objects which:

● have a greater mass
● are higher above ground
● are in a stronger gravitational field.

The gravitational field strength is sometimes known as the acceleration of free fall. Remember, gravitational field strength on Earth = 10 N/kg.

Falling Objects

A falling object converts gravitational potential energy to kinetic energy.

Consider a ball of mass 0.5 kg falling a distance of 15 m.

$$PE = mgh$$

$$= 0.5 \text{ kg} \times 10 \text{ N/kg} \times 15 \text{ m}$$

$$= 75 \text{ J}$$

Assuming no energy is lost, all of this energy is converted to kinetic energy.

$$KE = 75 \text{ J} = \frac{1}{2} mv^2$$

$$\frac{75 \text{ J}}{(\frac{1}{2} \, 0.5 \text{ kg})} = v^2$$

$$v^2 = 300$$

$$v = 17 \text{ m/s}$$

The speed of the ball after falling 15 m will be 17 m/s.

- Energy is transferred from one form to another; it can never be created or destroyed.
- Kinetic energy = $\frac{1}{2}$ × mass × velocity^2

Gravitational potential energy transferred = mass × gravitational field strength × change in height

QUESTIONS

QUICK TEST

1. What is the unit of energy?

2. What is the kinetic energy of a mass of 2.0 kg moving at a velocity of 3 m/s?

3. In what **three** ways can the gravitational potential energy of an object be increased?

EXAM PRACTICE

1. Look at the diagram of a rollercoaster ride. (Assume that gravitational field strength on Earth equals 10 N/kg.)

   a) What type of energy is gained as the car moves from point A to point B? **(1 mark)**

   b) Calculate the amount of energy gained if the mass of the car is 100 kg. **(1 mark)**

   c) Assuming all of this energy is converted into kinetic energy as the car moves from B to C, how much kinetic energy does the car have at C? **(1 mark)**

   d) Calculate the maximum speed at point C. **(2 marks)**

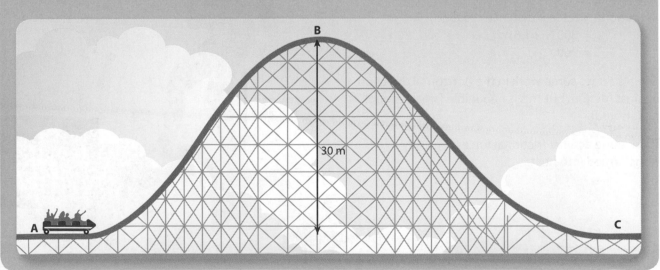

Work and Power

Work

Work done is equal to energy transferred. Work is done when a force moves an object.

One way of calculating the work done is to use the following equation:

> Work done = force × distance moved
> (in the direction
> of the force)

The amount of work done (joules) depends on:

- the size of the force in Newtons
- the distance moved in metres.

For example, work is done when a person is:

- lifting weights
- climbing stairs
- pulling a sledge
- pushing a shopping trolley.

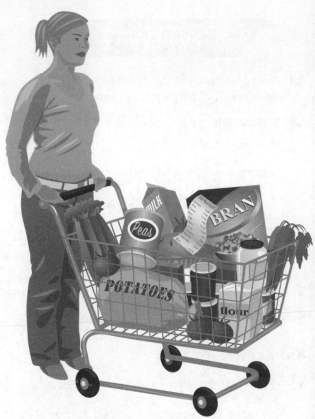

The girl opposite is running up stairs. She is doing work against her weight (the force directed downwards). This force is her mass, m, multiplied by the gravitational field strength, g. The distance in the direction of this force is the height of the stairs.

Work done = force × distance moved
$$= 600\,N \times 1.6\,m$$
$$= 960\,J$$

She also does some work in the horizontal direction against friction, but this is negligible (small enough to be ignored).

Work done against frictional forces is mainly transformed into heat.

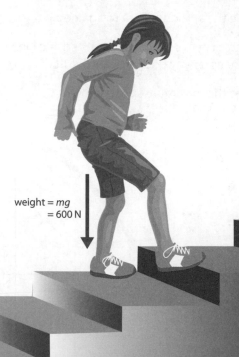

weight = mg
= 600 N

distance moved in the direction of the force = 1.6 m

Power

Power is a measurement of how quickly work is being done, and is measured in **watts** (W).

The faster work is done, the greater the power.

$$\text{Power} = \frac{\text{work done}}{\text{time taken}}$$

Example

Steve ran up a steep hill in 60 seconds. His weight was 800 N and the vertical height of the hill was 50 m. Work out the power.

$$\text{Power} = \frac{(800 \times 50)}{60} = \textbf{666.67 W}$$

Elastic Potential and Work

For an object that is able to recover its original shape, **elastic potential** is the energy stored in the object when work is done to change its shape.

Work Done in Lifting an Object

If an object is lifted a distance of h, the work done is equal to the weight $\times h$: weight $= mg$

So the work done in lifting an object is: work done $= mgh$

This is equal to the gain in gravitational potential energy ($PE = mgh$).

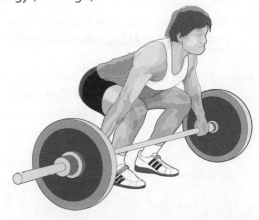

SUMMARY

- Work is done when a force moves an object.
- Work done = force × distance moved
- Power is how quickly work is being done, and is measured in watts.
- Power = $\frac{\text{work done}}{\text{time taken}}$
- When lifting an object:

Work done = mass × gravitational field strength × change in height

QUESTIONS

QUICK TEST

1. Define work.

2. Give **two** examples of when a person is doing work.

3. What work is done when an object is pushed with a force of 50 N for 2.0 m?

4. What is elastic potential energy?

EXAM PRACTICE

1. A crane lifts a load of 1500 kg 35 m into the air.

   a) Calculate the weight of this load. **(1 mark)**

   b) Calculate the work done by the crane. **(1 mark)**

   c) The crane lifts the load in 15 seconds. Calculate the power required. **(1 mark)**

   d) The crane next lifts a load of 5250 kg. How high would this load have to be lifted to give the same work as the original load? **(2 marks)**

Static Electricity

When some materials are rubbed together, **electrons** can be transferred from one material to the other.

- A build up of electrons creates a **negative charge**.
- A lack of electrons creates a **positive charge**.

Objects that have **opposite** charges will **attract**.

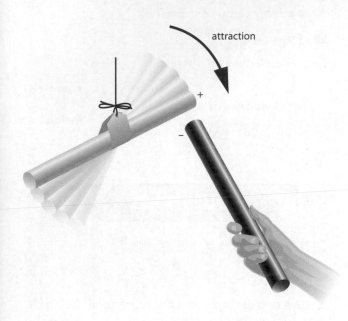

attraction

Objects that have the **same** charge will **repel**.

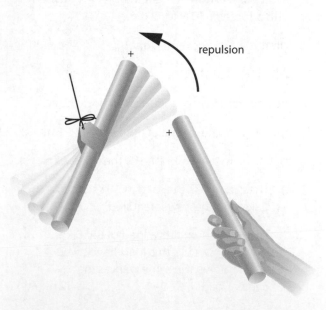

repulsion

Conductors and Insulators

Insulated materials can be charged by the transfer of electrons. If an object is connected to the ground by a conducting material, the charge flows away.

- **Conductor** – charge (electrons) can pass through.
- **Insulator** – charge cannot pass through.

When Static is Dangerous

If enough charge builds up, a spark may jump across the gap between the body and the earth or an earthed conductor.

- Aircraft fuel causes static as the fuel rubs against the pipe. A spark could ignite the fuel vapour. The aircraft and the tanker are earthed to avoid the charge building up.
- Lorries with inflammable gases and liquids are earthed before unloading.
- Lightning happens when charge builds up within a cloud. This can be caused by ice particles rubbing against the air. When the charge is large enough it leaps to another part of the cloud, or to the ground.

When Static is a Nuisance

Some situations do not involve enough charge to be dangerous. However, they can be a nuisance.

- Dirt and dust are attracted to television screens, monitors and plastic.
- Synthetic clothing clings.
- Cars are sometimes earthed to avoid shocks from car doors, caused by friction between you and the car.
- After walking across a floor covered with insulating material you may experience a shock if you touch water pipes, or some other earthed conductor.

Preventing Static Electricity

Some ways to prevent static shocks include:

- correct earthing
- insulating mats
- wearing rubber-soled shoes
- using anti-static sprays.

Uses of Static Electricity

- Photocopiers and laser printers use static to direct ink.
- Dust can be removed from chimneys by being attracted to a charged plate. Large particles form, falling when they are heavy enough or are shaken.
- Fingerprinting uses static electricity.
- Some dusters are designed to attract dust by static electricity.
- Doctors use static electricity to restart the heart.
- In paint spraying, paint is charged so that the droplets repel each other, giving a fine, even spray. A surface is given an opposite charge to the paint, ensuring an even coat and less waste.

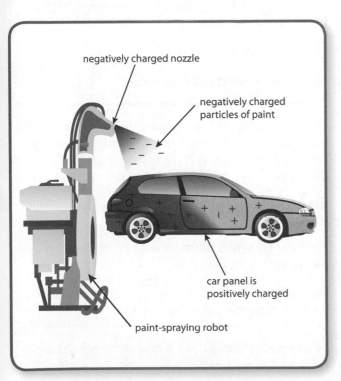

negatively charged nozzle

negatively charged particles of paint

car panel is positively charged

paint-spraying robot

SUMMARY

- A build up of electrons creates a negative charge. A lack of electrons creates a positive charge.
- A conductor allows charge to pass through it. An insulator prevents charge from passing through it.
- Static shocks can be prevented by ensuring that the charge doesn't earth through a person, e.g. by wearing rubber-soled shoes.

QUESTIONS

QUICK TEST

1. Define an electrical conductor.
2. Define an electrical insulator.
3. Why is an aircraft earthed when refuelling?
4. How can static be prevented?
5. Give an example of when static electricity can be a nuisance.

EXAM PRACTICE

1. A painter makes use of static electricity when spray painting a surface.

   a) Explain how static electricity ensures the surface is painted without any drips.
   (4 marks)

   b) Describe how workers carrying out the spraying might be at risk from static electricity.
   (1 mark)

   c) Explain how this risk could be reduced.
   (1 mark)

Electricity on the Move

Electric Current

Electric **current** is the movement of charge through a conductor. Current is measured in **Amps** or **Amperes** – it is equal to the amount of charge that flows every second. The unit of charge is the **Coulomb** (C).

This equation relates the amount of electrical charge that flows to current and time:

> Charge = current × time

The charged particles that flow in a wire are electrons, which have a **negative charge**. They flow from negative to positive.

Ions are positive particles left behind when the electrons move. We say that electric current is the flow of **positively** charged ions from positive to negative, but ions in a wire don't actually move.

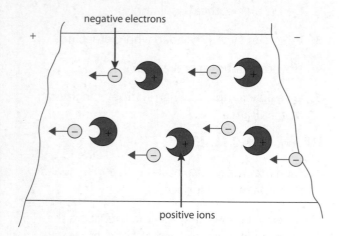

Providing a Potential Difference

Cells produce a flow of charge when a conducting wire is connected across their terminals, caused by the **potential difference** (p.d.) between the terminals. Potential difference is measured in **volts**; it is sometimes called **voltage**. The flow of current from a cell is always in one direction; it is called **direct current** or **DC**.

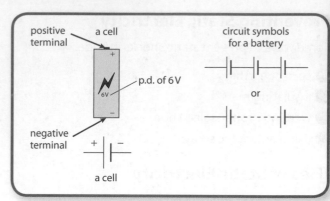

A **battery** is a number of cells connected in series. The number of hours a battery will last depends on its capacity in **Amp-hours** and the current it is supplying. Different appliances will take different currents from the same battery.

> $$\text{Hours} = \frac{\text{Amp-hours}}{\text{current supplied}}$$

Example
A battery is labelled 12 Amp-hours and it is used to supply 0.5 A to a CD player. How long will the battery last?

$$\frac{12\ \text{Amp-hours}}{0.5\ \text{A}} = 24\ \text{hours}$$

The battery will last for **24 hours**.

The mains supplies a potential difference of 230 V. The current supplied by the mains is called **alternating current** or **AC** because it continuously changes direction.

Energy

When electrical charge flows through a **resistor**, electrical **energy** is transformed into heat energy and the resistor heats up.

Energy transformed, potential difference and charge are related by the following equation:

> Energy transformed = potential difference × charge

Circuits

In order for a current to flow, a complete loop is required.

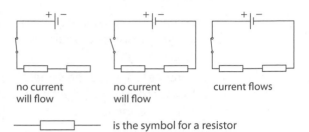

no current will flow   no current will flow   current flows

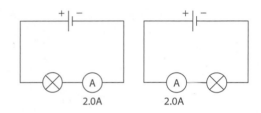 is the symbol for a resistor

Current is measured using an **ammeter**. The ammeter must be placed in **series** (next to) any other components. The current is the same at all points in a series circuit, so it can be placed either side of the component.

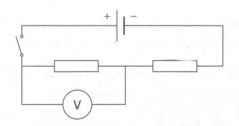

Potential difference is measured using a **voltmeter**. The voltmeter must be placed in **parallel** with the component that it is measuring.

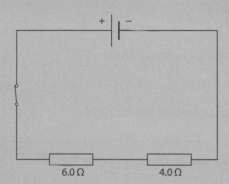

SUMMARY

- **Charge = current × time**
- **A cell produces direct current.**
- **The number of hours a battery can power a device can be calculated using:**

  $$\text{Hours} = \frac{\text{Amp-hours}}{\text{current supplied}}$$

- $$\frac{\text{Energy}}{\text{transformed}} = \frac{\text{potential}}{\text{difference}} \times \text{charge}$$

- **Ammeters measure current and voltmeters measure potential difference.**

QUESTIONS

QUICK TEST

1. How is current measured?

2. What charge flows per second if the current is 5.0 A?

3. Are the following statements true or false?

   a) Electrons have a negative charge.

   b) Electrons flow from positive to negative.

   c) Ions in a wire flow from positive to negative.

   d) Current is said to flow from positive to negative.

EXAM PRACTICE

1.

a) In the above circuit, electricity flows from positive to negative. Add arrows to the circuit to show the direction of current flow. **(1 mark)**

b) Add an ammeter to the circuit to measure the current through the resistors. **(1 mark)**

c) Add a voltmeter that will measure the potential difference across the 4.0 Ω resistor. **(1 mark)**

d) What will happen if the switch is opened? **(1 mark)**

2. A charge of 2000 Coulombs is passed through a circuit in 15 seconds. What is the current in the circuit? **(2 marks)**

Resistance

Resistance is a measure of how easy or how difficult it is for electricity to flow through a material.

Current passes easily through copper wire because it has a **low resistance**. However, current does not pass so easily through a filament lamp. The filament lamp has a **higher resistance**. More energy is needed to push the electrons through the filament wire in the lamp. This energy is converted to heat (and light) in the lamp. Components with a higher resistance give off more heat.

Calculating Resistance

Resistance is measured in **Ohms** (Ω). The resistance of a component is found using the following equation:

> Resistance = $\dfrac{\text{potential difference}}{\text{current}}$
>
> Resistance is measured in ohms (Ω)
>
> Potential difference (voltage) is measured in volts (V)
>
> Current is measured in amps (A)

In the circuit below, there is a potential difference across the component of 12.0 V and a current through it of 3.0 A.

Resistance = $\dfrac{12.0\,\text{V}}{3.0\,\text{A}}$ = 4.0 Ω

- If the potential difference remained the same, a component with a higher resistance would have a *lower* current passing through it.
- If the potential difference remained the same, a component with a lower resistance would have a *higher* current passing through it.
- For a given resistor, current increases as p.d. increases.
- For a given resistor, current decreases as p.d. decreases.

In **series**, the total resistance equals the sum of the individual resistances.

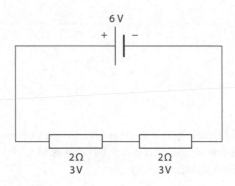

6 V
+ –

2Ω
3 V

2Ω
3 V

- There is the same current in each component.
- The p.d. of the supply is shared by the components.

In **parallel**, the total resistance is less than each of the individual resistors.

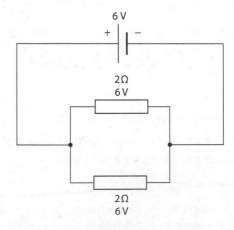

6 V
+ –

2Ω
6 V

2Ω
6 V

- The p.d. across each component is the same.
- The current is shared by the components.

component

A

ammeter 3.0 A

V

voltmeter 12.0 V

Changing Resistance

The resistance of some resistors can change. Resistors are usually made from wire where the resistance increases when:

- the wire is longer
- the wire gets hotter
- the wire is thinner.

A **variable resistor** is a device with a control to vary its resistance. The symbol for a variable resistor is:

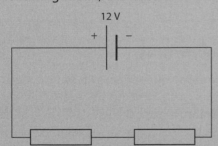

SUMMARY

- Resistance is a measure of how easy or difficult it is for electricity to flow through a material.
- Resistance is measured in Ohms.
- $\text{Resistance} = \dfrac{\text{potential difference}}{\text{current}}$
- Resistance can be increased by making a wire longer or by increasing the temperature of the wire.

QUESTIONS

QUICK TEST

1. Find the resistance of a component with a p.d. of 6.0 V and a current of 4.0 A.

2. A resistor is replaced with a resistor of higher resistance. How will the current in the circuit change?

3. What is the circuit symbol for a variable resistor?

4. How would decreasing the length of a resistance wire change its resistance?

EXAM PRACTICE

1. In the following circuit, the resistors each have resistance of 5 Ω.

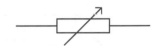

   a) What is the total resistance?   (1 mark)

   b) What is the current through each resistor?   (1 mark)

   c) What is the p.d. across each resistor?   (1 mark)

   d) How could both resistors be arranged so that the total resistance is less than 5 Ω?   (1 mark)

Electrical Power

Electrical power is a measure of the rate at which a device uses energy.

An appliance that uses more energy per second has more power. Power is measured in **watts** (W). An appliance that uses 1 joule of energy in 1 second has a power of 1 watt.

A light bulb with a power of 60 W uses 60 J of energy per second. A light bulb with a power of 100 W uses 100 J of energy per second.

100 W bulb   **60 W bulb**

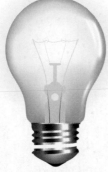   

100 J of energy used per second   60 J of energy used per second

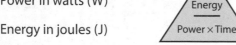

Power = $\dfrac{\text{energy}}{\text{time}}$

Power in watts (W)

Energy in joules (J)

Time in seconds (s)

Energy
Power × Time

Example
A hairdryer of 1200 W (1.2 kW) is used for 2 minutes. How much energy is used?

Energy = power × time

= 1200 W × 120 s

= 144 000 J = **144 kJ**

Calculating Electrical Power

Power is calculated using the following equation:

Electrical power = potential difference (voltage) × current

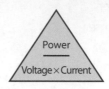

Power
Voltage × Current

Examples
1. A games console operates on a voltage of 230 V and a current of 0.8 A. Calculate its power.

   Power = voltage × current

   = 230 V × 0.8 A

   = **184 W**

2. An electric drill operates on a voltage of 230 V and has a power of 400 W.
   Calculate the current drawn by the drill.

   Current = $\dfrac{\text{power}}{\text{voltage}}$

   = $\dfrac{400\,\text{W}}{230\,\text{V}}$

   = **1.7 A**

Domestic Bills

The standard unit for energy is joules. A typical appliance uses a large number of joules. The hairdryer in the example opposite uses 144 000 J in just 2 minutes!

For domestic bills, it is more convenient to use a larger unit. The **kilowatt-hour** is a larger unit of **energy**.

An appliance with a power of 1000 W (1 kW) switched on for 1 hour uses 1 kilowatt-hour of energy. (Compare this to an appliance with a power of 1 W switched on for 1 s which uses 1 J of energy.)

Example

A fridge of 1.5 kW is switched on for 8 hours. How many kWh does it use?

Energy = power × time

= 1.5 kW × 8 hours

= **12 kWh**

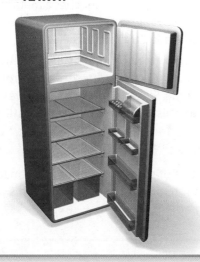

Electricity companies refer to kWh as **units** of energy.

The cost can be calculated by multiplying the number of units by the cost of a unit.

> Cost = number of units (kWh) × cost of a unit

QUESTIONS

QUICK TEST

1. A personal stereo produces 1.5 J of sound energy per second. What is its power?

2. a) Calculate the energy in joules used by a 2000 W kettle in 2 minutes.

   b) Calculate the energy in kWh used by a 2000 W kettle in 2 minutes.

3. A lamp is marked with the following information: 12 W, 2.5 V. Calculate the current through the lamp.

4. An electricity company charges 12p for each unit of electricity used. Calculate the cost of operating a 2 kW heater for 4 hours.

EXAM PRACTICE

1. A table lamp has three bulbs, each of 40 W.

   a) Find the energy in joules and in kWh used by each bulb per hour. **(2 marks)**

   b) If each unit costs 10p, find the cost of lighting the table lamp for 24 hours. **(2 marks)**

   c) It is suggested that the bulbs are replaced with low energy bulbs of 5 W each, giving out the same light, but less heat. How much energy in kWh is used by each bulb per hour? **(1 mark)**

   d) Calculate the kWh used by the lamp in 24 hours with low energy bulbs, assuming each unit costs 10p, and find the cost of lighting the table lamp for 24 hours. **(2 marks)**

Electricity at Home

Plugs

A plug has three wires: **live**, **neutral** and **earth**.

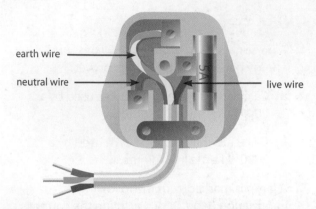

earth wire

neutral wire

live wire

	Colour	Function
Live	brown	alternating between positive and negative voltage
Neutral	blue	completes the circuit, stays at zero voltage
Earth	green and yellow	safety wire

Safe Electricity

Too much current in a wire causes overheating and can cause a fire.

Some ways of improving safety when using electricity are listed here:

- A **fuse** is a short piece of thin wire placed in a circuit that melts with high current, breaking the circuit. The live wire must be connected through the fuse. The power equation can be used to determine the size fuse a device needs. For example, a kettle of 2000 W uses mains voltage of 230 V.

  Power = current × voltage

  $$\text{Current} = \frac{2000\,\text{W}}{230\,\text{V}} = 8.7\,\text{A}$$

  The fuse must have a higher rating than the current flowing through the appliance, so this appliance needs a 10 A fuse.

- **Residual current circuit breakers** (RCCBs) improve the safety of a device by disconnecting a circuit automatically whenever it detects a difference in current between the neutral and the live wire.

- An **earth wire** is a safety wire that connects the metal parts of a device to earth and stops the device becoming dangerous to touch if there is a loose wire. If a wire works loose and touches a metal part of the device, a large current flows to earth, blowing the fuse or activating the circuit breaker.

- Many modern devices are insulated with a plastic case, which insulates the user from any wiring faults. Since the wires themselves are also insulated, this is known as **double insulation**.

Changing Resistance

The resistance of some components is constant at a constant temperature. On a graph this gives a constant gradient.

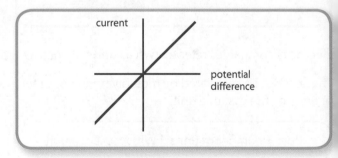

current

potential difference

The resistance of a **filament lamp** increases with more current as the lamp gets hotter. This is due to increased kinetic energy causing more collisions between the electrons and ions. This increases the ions' vibration, causing the increase in temperature and resistance.

The symbol for a lamp is:

or

As the resistance increases with current, the gradient in a current–potential difference graph decreases to reflect this.

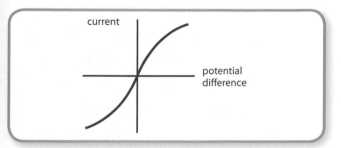

The current through a **diode** flows in one direction only. It has a very high resistance in the reverse direction. The symbol for a diode is:

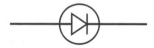

On a graph, no current flows in the reverse direction.

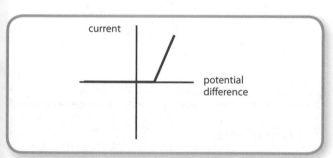

A **light dependent resistor** (LDR) has a high resistance in the dark and a low resistance in the light. It is used to detect light or switch a lamp on automatically in the dark. The symbol for an LDR is:

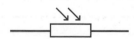

A **thermistor** has a high resistance when cold and a low resistance when hot. It is used to detect temperature change for a thermostat. The symbol for a thermistor is:

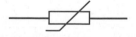

SUMMARY

- Plugs have three wires: live (brown), neutral (blue) and earth (green and yellow).
- Fuses are wires that melt with high current.
- As the current through a filament lamp increases, the resistance increases.
- A diode has a very high resistance in the reverse direction.
- An LDR has a high resistance in the dark and a low resistance in the light.
- A thermistor has a high resistance when cold and a low resistance when warm.

QUESTIONS

QUICK TEST

1. A hairdryer has an earth wire and a fuse. Explain how this protects the user.

2. What is an RCCB and what is its purpose?

3. How does the resistance of a filament lamp change with current?

EXAM PRACTICE

1. In a plug, what must the live wire be connected through? **(1 mark)**

2. Explain why a hairdryer that is double insulated does not require an earth wire. **(2 marks)**

3. A thermistor is placed in a beaker of crushed ice. What happens to its resistance? **(1 mark)**

4. Suggest a suitable fuse for a vacuum cleaner of power 900 W and voltage 230 V. **(2 marks)**

5. Increasing the current through a bulb increases its resistance. Use kinetic energy to explain why this occurs.

   The quality of written communication will be assessed in your answer to this question.
   (6 marks)

Controlling Voltage

Potential Dividers

Resistors can be used in a circuit to control the voltage in a number of ways.

Two resistors arranged in series can be arranged as a **potential divider**, where:

$$V_{out} = V_{in} \left(\frac{R_2}{R_1 + R_2} \right)$$

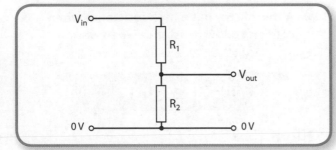

If the input voltage is 12 V and $R_1 = 4\,\Omega$ and $R_2 = 2\,\Omega$, the output voltage would be:

$$12V \left(\frac{2\Omega}{(4\Omega + 2\Omega)} \right) = 4V$$

If one of the resistors is replaced with a variable resistor, then the output voltage can be adjusted.

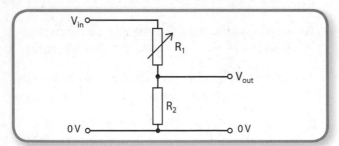

If one of the resistors is replaced with a thermistor, the output signal can be used as a sensor of heat.

The resistance of a thermistor is high when it is cold, so the voltage across the thermistor is high. In the following circuit, the output voltage across R_2 is low when cold. When hot, the thermistor's resistance decreases, producing a higher output voltage.

If R_2 is replaced with a thermistor instead of R_1, then the output is reversed.

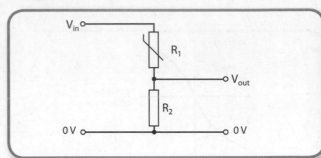

If one of the resistors is replaced with an LDR, the output signal can be used as a sensor of light.

In the following circuit, R_2 has been replaced with an LDR. When it is dark the LDR has a high resistance, and when light it has a low resistance. The output voltage is high when it is dark and low when it is light.

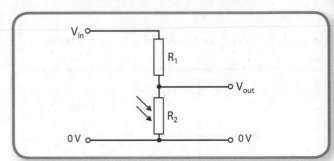

Rectification

A **diode** can be used to control voltage. A diode only allows electricity to pass through it in one direction. If an alternating current (AC) passes through a diode it becomes a direct current, although it is not smooth like the direct current from a cell.

This is called **half wave rectification**.

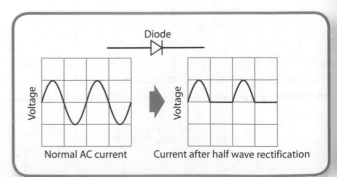

Normal AC current   Current after half wave rectification

A bridge circuit with four diodes produces an AC trace like the one below. This is called **full wave rectification**.

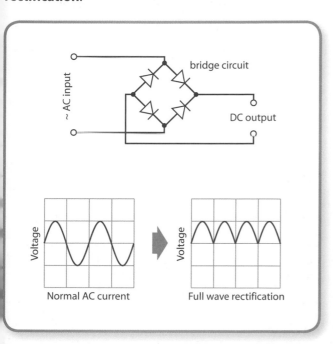

bridge circuit

~ AC input

DC output

Voltage — Normal AC current

Voltage — Full wave rectification

Capacitors

Many devices need a more constant voltage supply. A **capacitor** can be used to smooth out current that has been rectified in a bridge circuit. The symbol for a capacitor is:

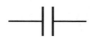

A capacitor is a device that stores charge. When a current flows in a circuit containing an uncharged capacitor, charge is stored and the potential difference, (p.d.) across the capacitor increases.

If a conductor is connected across a charged capacitor, the current flows. As the capacitor discharges, the p.d. across it and the current flowing decreases.

SUMMARY

● Two resistors in series can be arranged as a potential divider.

● If an alternating current passes through a diode, it undergoes half wave rectification.

● A bridge circuit with four diodes can cause full wave rectification.

● A capacitor is used to smooth out current that has been rectified in a bridge circuit.

QUESTIONS

QUICK TEST

1. An AC supply is passed through a single diode. Sketch the shape of the output voltage.

2. Name the process in question 1.

3. Name the process when four diodes are used in a bridge circuit.

4. What is the circuit symbol for a capacitor?

5. Why might a capacitor be included in a bridge circuit?

EXAM PRACTICE

1. A voltmeter is wired across a capacitor. What would happen to the value shown by the voltmeter when:

   a) the capacitor was uncharged and connected to a circuit with a battery? Explain your answer. **(2 marks)**

   b) the capacitor was charged and it was placed in a circuit with a battery? Explain your answer. **(2 marks)**

2. Explain how a potential divider could be set up to give a high voltage output when it is cold. **(4 marks)**

Electronic Applications

Logic Gates

Many electrical devices rely on some form of **logic circuit**, including computers, washing machines and car ignitions.

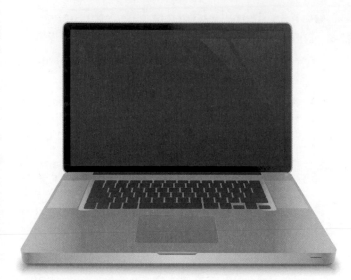

The input signal for a logic gate is either a high voltage (about 5V) or a low voltage (about 0V). A high signal is referred to as 1 and a low signal as 0.

NOT Gate

The most simple logic gate is a NOT gate that reverses the input. An input of 0 gives an output of 1 and an input of 1 gives an output of 0.

The table below is known as a **truth table**.

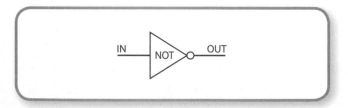

Input	Output
1	0
0	1

AND Gate

An AND gate has two inputs. It gives an output of 1 when both the first and the second input are 1. Otherwise the output is 0.

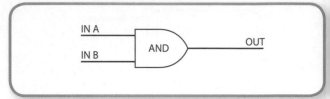

Input A	Input B	Output
0	1	0
0	0	0
1	0	0
1	1	1

OR Gate

An OR gate has two inputs. It gives an output of 1 when either the first input or the second input or both inputs are 1.

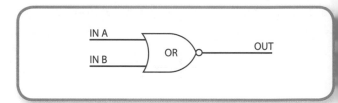

Input A	Input B	Output
0	0	0
0	1	1
1	0	1
1	1	1

An OR gate could be used to control the courtesy light in a car, so that it comes on if the driver's door or the passenger's door or both doors are open.

NAND Gate

A NAND gate has two inputs, and its output is the opposite of an AND gate.

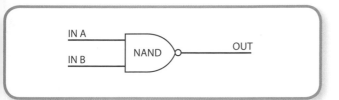

Input A	Input B	Output
0	0	1
0	1	1
1	0	1
1	1	0

NOR Gate

A NOR gate has two inputs, and its output is the opposite of an OR gate.

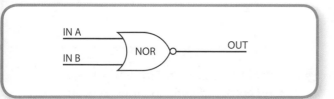

Input A	Input B	Output
0	0	1
0	1	0
1	0	0
1	1	0

SUMMARY

- A logic gate either has a high voltage (1) or a low voltage input (0).

- NOT gates only give an output of 1 if the input is 0.

- AND gates only give an output of 1 if both inputs are 1.

- OR gates give an output of 1 if either input is 1.

- A NAND gate gives the opposite output to an AND gate, and a NOR gate gives the opposite output to an OR gate.

QUESTIONS

QUICK TEST

1. Draw a NOT gate.

2. Write the truth table for a NOT gate.

3. Draw a NOR gate.

4. Write the truth table for a NOR gate.

5. Suggest a use for an OR gate.

EXAM PRACTICE

1. What are the two input signals for a logic gate? **(2 marks)**

2. Complete the truth table below for an OR gate. **(4 marks)**

Input A	Input B	Output
1	0	
0		1
1	1	
		0

3. How would a NOR gate truth table differ from the one shown above? **(2 marks)**

Producing Electricity

Generators

Electricity is generated in a power station by rotating a magnet near a coil of wire (or by rotating a coil of wire near a magnet). This produces a current in the coil of wire and is called the **dynamo effect**.

Dynamos or generators produce a current that changes direction every time the magnet turns. This is called **alternating current** or **AC**. The current supplied to our homes is AC.

The current and the voltage of a dynamo can be increased by:

- increasing the strength of the magnet
- increasing the number of turns in the coil of wire
- increasing the speed of rotation of the magnet.

AC and DC current can be displayed on an oscilloscope:

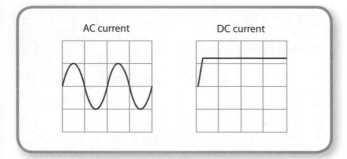

Measuring Current

The current in a circuit is measured using an **ammeter**. The ammeter must be placed in the circuit in **series** (next to) any other components. The current is the same at all points in a series circuit, so it can be placed either side of the component.

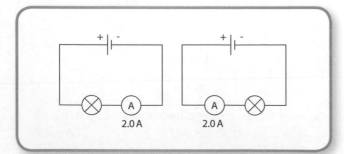

The National Grid

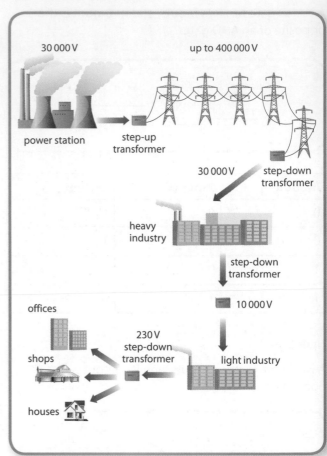

- The National Grid distributes electricity to consumers at different voltages using **step-up** and **step-down transformers**. Consumers include homes, factories, offices, schools and farms.

- It is more efficient to transmit electricity at a much higher voltage than is required by consumers. Increasing the voltage decreases the current in the transmission cables. The cables lose less heat energy when the current is lower.

- Overhead cables are the cheapest way of transmitting electricity. Underground cables are more expensive, but do not spoil the landscape.

- The National Grid allows electricity to be distributed from areas where consumption is low to areas where there is high consumption.

- Electricity is supplied to our homes at 230 V.

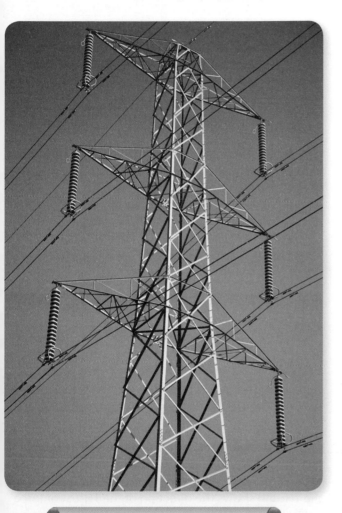

QUICK TEST

1. Why does the National Grid transmit electricity at high voltages?

2. Give an example of a 'high voltage'.

3. Give **one** advantage of using underground cables to distribute electricity.

EXAM PRACTICE

1. The diagram shows a simple generator. When the coil is rotated, a current flows and lights the lamp.

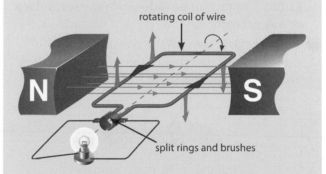

rotating coil of wire

N   S

split rings and brushes

a) Give **three** ways of increasing the current in the coil. **(3 marks)**

b) Is the current produced AC or DC? **(1 mark)**

c) Explain the difference between AC and DC. **(2 marks)**

d) Add to the diagram an ammeter that would measure the current passing through the lamp. **(1 mark)**

SUMMARY

- The dynamo effect (rotating a magnet near a coil of wire) produces an electric current.

- Current can be either AC or DC.

- An ammeter is used to measure current. It is wired In series in a circuit.

- The National Grid uses step-up transformers to increase voltage to distribute electricity through power lines.

- Step-down transformers are used to decrease voltage, to make electricity safe to use in our homes.

Transformers and Motors

Transformers

Transformers change the voltage of an **alternating** electricity supply.

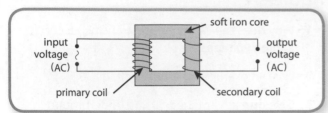

- A **primary coil** is an electric cable wrapped around a soft iron core. It is connected to an input power supply providing **alternating** current.
- The alternating current creates a **changing** magnetic field in the soft iron.
- The changing magnetic field in the soft iron core causes a voltage to be **induced** in the **secondary** or **output coil**.
- The number of turns of the primary and the secondary coil determines the change in voltage according to the following equation:

$$\frac{\text{primary or input voltage}}{\text{secondary or output voltage}} = \frac{\text{number of turns on primary coil}}{\text{number of turns on secondary coil}}$$

Example

On a transformer, the primary coil has 6 turns on it and the secondary coil has 3 turns. The input voltage on the primary coil is 100 V. What is the output voltage?

$$\frac{6 \text{ turns on primary coil}}{3 \text{ turns on secondary coil}} = 2$$

$$2 = \frac{100 \text{ V}}{\text{output voltage}}$$

$$\text{Output voltage} = \frac{100 \text{ V}}{2}$$

$$\text{Output voltage} = \textbf{50 V}$$

- A **step-up transformer** increases the voltage (has more turns on the secondary coil than the primary coil) and a **step-down transformer** decreases the voltage (has more turns on the primary coil than the secondary coil).

Motors

A current-carrying wire has a circular **magnetic field** around it. The field is made up of concentric circles. When a current-carrying straight wire is placed in a magnetic field, it experiences a force and can move.

The direction of this force can be found using **Fleming's left-hand rule**. A hand is held with two fingers and the thumb perpendicular.

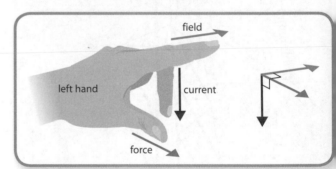

The First finger is pointed in the direction of the Field, the seCond finger in the direction of the Current and the THumb shows the direction of the THrust or force.

Motors take electrical energy and transform it into kinetic (movement) energy.

This simple motor runs on DC (direct current) from a battery. The current flows in the coil, which experiences a turning effect caused by the magnetic field.

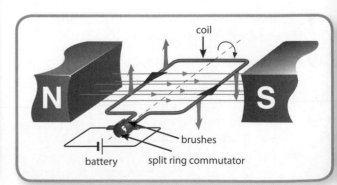

The forces on the coil can only pull the coil half a turn because the forces then pull the wrong way. A motor allows the coil to continue to turn by changing the direction of the forces. It does this by changing the direction of the current – as the coil spins, the commutator spins, but the brushes remain in the same place, changing the direction of the current every half turn.

A stronger turning effect is produced by:

- increasing the number of turns on the coil
- increasing the current
- using a stronger magnet.

Motors are found in a variety of everyday applications such as washing machines, CD players and electric drills.

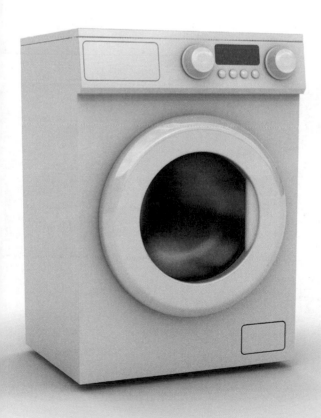

QUESTIONS

QUICK TEST

1. The input voltage of a transformer is 230V and the primary coil has 1200 turns. If the secondary coil has 100 turns, what is the output voltage?

2. Give **three** ways of increasing the turning effect of a motor.

EXAM PRACTICE

1. The diagram shows a transformer.

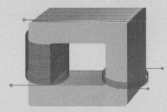

a) Label the primary coil and the secondary coil in the diagram. **(2 marks)**

b) Is this a step-up transformer or a step-down transformer? **(1 mark)**

c) The transformer has an input voltage of 600 V. The primary coil has 50 turns and the secondary coil has 4 turns. Calculate the output voltage across the secondary coil. **(2 marks)**

Electricity in the World

Everyday Use

Some examples of everyday devices designed to bring about particular energy transformations are listed below:

- A hairdryer converts electrical energy to kinetic energy and heat.
- A microphone converts sound (kinetic energy of the air) to electrical energy.
- A light bulb converts electrical energy to light and heat.

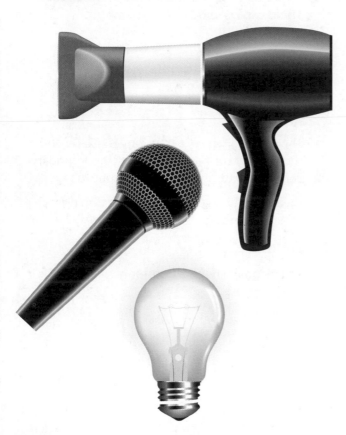

The development of the use of electricity and telecommunications has had a great impact on society.

Here are some of the ways that things have changed over time:

- Electric circuits have become much smaller, greatly increasing the processing speed of computers, and allowing development of many new applications.

- The electric telephone has replaced rotary dialling with touch-tone dialling, which greatly increases the capacity and quality of the network. Digital signalling has replaced analogue, allowing multiplexing (sending many signals at once).
- Superconductivity is the decrease in resistance to almost zero in certain materials at extremely low temperatures. The technology is used to make very powerful electromagnets used in MRI machines and particle accelerators.
- The use of ICT in collecting and displaying data for analysis has improved reliability and validity of data, and encourages faster development of new technology.
- Maglev trains suspend, propel and direct trains using magnetic forces and magnetic levitation from electromagnets attached to the train. The decreased friction allows trains to reach speeds of nearly 600 km/h.

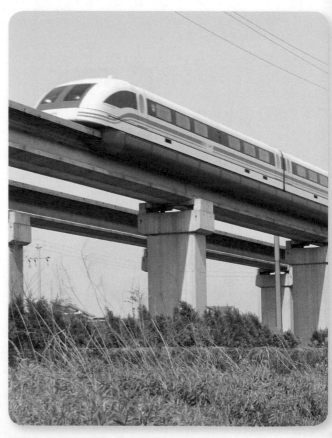

Analogue and Digital Signals

Analogue signals have a continuously variable value.

Digital signals are either on or off.

It is easier to remove noise from a digital signal than an analogue signal as it's either on or off.

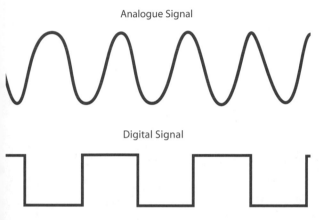

Analogue Signal

Digital Signal

Lasers

Lasers produce a beam of monochromatic (single colour) light.

Lasers can be used…

- for industrial cutting
- for surgical and dental treatment
- in weapon guidance
- for laser light shows
- in CD/DVD players.

A laser in a CD player reflects from the surface, which contains digital information in a pattern of pits.

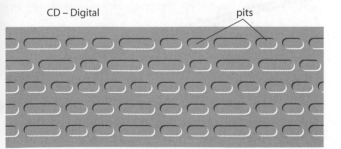

CD – Digital   pits

SUMMARY

- Devices convert electrical energy to many different types of energy.

- Electronic signals can be analogue or digital.

- Analogue signals have a continuously variable value. Digital signals are either on or off.

- Lasers produce a beam of monochromatic light.

QUESTIONS

QUICK TEST

1. How has the size of electric circuits affected computers?

2. What is multiplexing?

3. How can a maglev train reach speeds of almost 600 km/h?

4. What is superconductivity?

EXAM PRACTICE

1. Describe the difference between analogue and digital signals. **(2 marks)**

2. Is interference easier to remove from a digital or an analogue signal? Explain your answer. **(2 marks)**

3. Describe how data is stored on a CD and how this data is read by a laser. **(4 marks)**

Harnessing Energy 1

Fossil Fuels

Most of our energy comes from **fossil fuels** such as oil, coal or gas. Fossil fuels are a **non-renewable** energy source used to generate electrical energy. They release gases into the environment that pollute the atmosphere.

Fossil fuels are burned. The heat generated is used to boil water in a boiler to produce steam. This steam is used to turn a turbine, which is connected to a generator. The generator then generates electricity.

The energy change when burning fossil fuels is from **chemical energy** to **heat** to **kinetic energy** (in a turbine that turns a generator) to **electrical energy**.

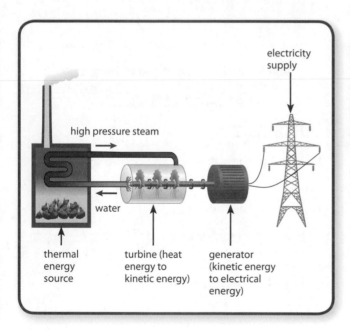

high pressure steam

electricity supply

water

thermal energy source

turbine (heat energy to kinetic energy)

generator (kinetic energy to electrical energy)

Renewable Energy Sources

Energy can be harnessed from sources such as the Sun, the force of the wind and moving water. These energy sources are **renewable**. They require no fuel and release no polluting gases into the environment.

However, there are often difficulties associated with renewable energy sources, including other problems for the environment. Many renewable energy sources are also unreliable and expensive. Many people think we should aim to reduce the amount of energy we use in our homes and workplaces.

Wind Power

A wind farm is a collection of generators driven by wind turbines. The generators are used to produce energy.

There are problems associated with wind farms:

- They require large areas of land.
- They are dependent on wind speed.
- They produce noise, which can disturb wildlife.
- They can be expensive to build.
- They change the view of the landscape.

The energy change is from **kinetic energy** of the wind to **electrical energy**.

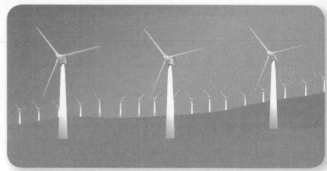

Waves and Tides

Energy can be harnessed from the rise and fall of water due to waves and tides. The **kinetic energy** of the water can be used to drive turbines, which generate **electrical energy**.

A disadvantage is that wave and tidal barrages are very difficult to build.

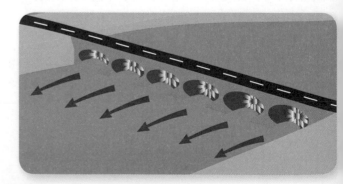

Hydroelectric Power

To generate hydroelectric power, rivers and rain fill up a high reservoir behind a dam. The water is released and used to drive turbines that generate electricity. The energy changes are **gravitational potential energy** (of the water) to **kinetic energy** (of the water) to **kinetic energy** (of the turbine) to **electrical energy**.

Harnessing energy from water can disturb natural habitats. Tidal barrages and dams flood areas and remove water from other areas artificially.

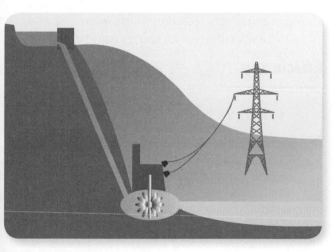

Geothermal Energy

In some volcanic areas, hot water and steam rise to the surface. Water can also be pumped down to hot rocks and steam is generated. The steam can be used to drive turbines. The energy change is from **heat** to **kinetic energy** to **electrical energy**.

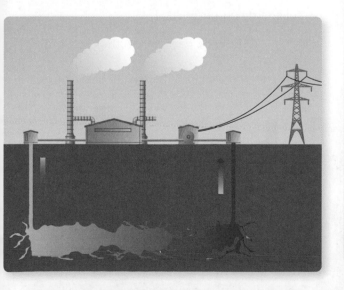

SUMMARY

- Fossil fuels can be burned to generate electricity. However, this creates gases that pollute the atmosphere.

- Wind, waves, tidal power, hydroelectric and geothermal power are all examples of renewable energy sources.

- Whilst renewable energy sources are less polluting than fossil fuels, they all have some environmental impact.

QUESTIONS

QUICK TEST

1. Name the energy changes that take place in a coal-fired power station burning fossil fuels.

2. Give **three** renewable energy sources.

3. Name an advantage of hydroelectric power.

4. Name a disadvantage of hydroelectric power.

5. Name the energy change that takes place when using geothermal energy.

EXAM PRACTICE

1. Complete the following sentences.

   Natural gas is a .... fuel. In a gas-fired power station, gas is burned to heat .... in a .... This forms steam that is used to turn a .... The .... is connected to a .... that produces electricity. **(3 marks)**

2. Local residents often protest when there are plans to build wind farms near their homes. Give three concerns that local residents might have. **(3 marks)**

3. What are the similarities and differences between wave power and hydroelectric power? **(3 marks)**

Harnessing Energy 2

Biomass

Fuels made from animal or plant material are known as **biomass**. Like fossil fuels they are burned and the heat energy produced is used to make steam to drive a turbine. Producing biomass requires a large area of land.

Solar Power

Solar cells convert energy from the Sun into electricity. **Solar panels** use infrared radiation from the Sun to heat water.

Solar cells are very expensive and sunshine is not reliable in many locations.

Nuclear Power

Nuclear power can also be used to produce electricity. Heat generated from nuclear fission is used to create steam that drives a turbine. Nuclear power is non-renewable.

Environmental Issues

- Power stations that burn fuel put carbon dioxide gas (CO_2) into the atmosphere. The gases act like a greenhouse and trap energy from the Sun, which may cause **global warming**. This **greenhouse effect** is important – without it our world would not be warm enough for life to exist. Extra warming, however, could cause problems for humans, plants and animals. Deforestation and increased CO_2 also contribute to global warming.

- Some power stations give off other gases such as sulfur dioxide, which can cause **acid rain**. Acid rain damages buildings, stone and trees.

- A radioactive leak could cause damage to humans and wildlife for many years. Radioactive dust can be carried by the wind for thousands of kilometres.

- The ozone layer protects the Earth from ultraviolet radiation, and pollution from CFCs is depleting the ozone layer.

- Dust from volcanoes reflects radiation from the Sun back into space, which causes cooling. Dust from factories reflects radiation from the ground and particularly cities, which causes warming.

Efficiency

$$\text{Efficiency} = \frac{\text{useful energy output}}{\text{total energy input}} \times 100\%$$

All devices waste energy; this energy is usually lost as heat to the surroundings.

For example, your body uses energy. If you run up a flight of stairs, you may use 2000 J of energy. This energy comes from stored energy in the food you eat. However, only about 15% of this energy is transferred to the movement in your muscles. The rest is wasted as heat in your body and heat to the surroundings. So about 300 J would be transferred to kinetic energy and 1700 J to heat.

Total energy input = 2000 J

Useful energy output = 300 J

$$\text{Efficiency} = \frac{300}{2000} \times 100\%$$

$$= 15\%$$

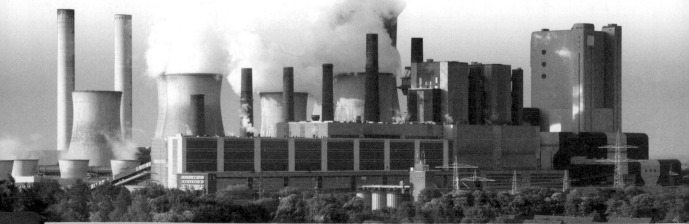

The **sankey diagram** below shows the energy efficiency for a person running up a flight of stairs.

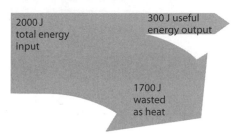

Here are some typical efficiencies of other devices:

An electric motor   80%
A petrol engine   25%
A candle   5%

A petrol engine loses 75% of its energy as heat. This is why cars need cooling systems.

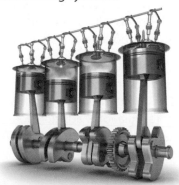

SUMMARY

● **Burning fuels releases carbon dioxide. This leads to the greenhouse effect, which in turn could cause climate change.**

● **The burning of some fuels releases sulfur dioxide, which can lead to acid rain.**

● **Nuclear power stations could suffer from radiation leaks. This could have a devastating effect on the local environment and human population.**

● **Efficiency = $\dfrac{\text{useful energy output}}{\text{total energy input}} \times 100\%$**

QUESTIONS

QUICK TEST

1. State **one** disadvantage of biomass.

2. What chemical causes acid rain?

3. What gas is said to cause the greenhouse effect and global warming?

4. Which gases damage the ozone layer?

5. How does dust from factories affect the climate?

EXAM PRACTICE

1. a) If a car burns 4000 J of energy but 3000 J is lost, what is its efficiency?   **(1 mark)**

    b) How is energy lost from the car?   **(1 mark)**

2. Kim uses a hairdryer. Some of the energy is wasted as sound. The sankey diagram shows the total energy input and the output.

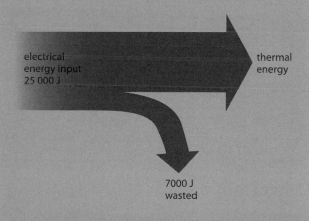

    a) Calculate the useful energy output. **(1 mark)**

    b) Calculate the efficiency of the hairdryer.   **(2 marks)**

Keeping Warm

Heat travels from hot places to cold places. This generally results in hot things cooling down (losing their heat) and cold things heating up (gaining heat). A warm house in winter can be kept warm using **insulation**.

Heat can move in three ways:

- **Conduction**
- **Convection**
- **Radiation**

Conduction

Conduction involves the heat moving from one particle to another, usually in a solid. Some materials are better thermal conductors than others. Metal is a good conductor since it allows the heat to travel through it quickly (because the electrons are mobile). Plastic and wood are poor conductors, so are known as insulators. Most liquids are also poor conductors, so act as insulators. Many good thermal insulators have pockets of air trapped in them, as air is a very poor conductor of heat.

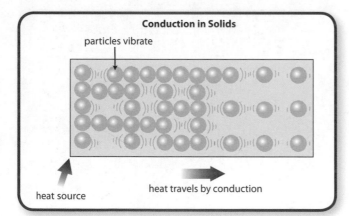

Conduction in Solids

particles vibrate

heat travels by conduction

heat source

Convection

Convection involves the movement of particles in a gas or a liquid. Thermals are areas of hot air rising (cooler air sinks). The air circulates in a **convection current**.

Hot air rises because it expands and becomes less dense (has less mass per unit volume). Cool air sinks because it is more dense.

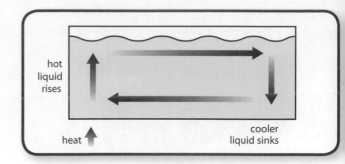

hot liquid rises

heat

cooler liquid sinks

Heat circulates from a heater around a room by convection currents. Convection cannot take place in a solid since the particles are not free to move.

Heat transfer by convection can be reduced by trapping air, such as in double glazing.

Radiation

Radiation is the transfer of heat energy by **infrared electromagnetic waves**. All bodies emit and absorb thermal radiation. The hotter a body is, the more energy it radiates.

Dark, matt objects absorb more radiation than light, shiny objects. This results in dark objects heating up more and emitting more radiation. Radiation does not require particles, so it can travel through a vacuum. This is how the Sun's energy reaches Earth.

Insulating Houses

Here are some ways that a house can be insulated. You will notice that many of them trap air and, therefore, reduce heat transfer by convection.

- Double glazing traps air between two layers of glass.
- Curtains trap air.
- Loft insulation traps air, which stops hot air rising and escaping through the roof.
- Cavity walls trap air or cavities in walls are often filled with insulation, which further reduces the movement of the air.
- Draught proofing.
- Reflective foil on or in walls reduces heat loss by radiation.
- Insulation (lagging) around the hot water tank.

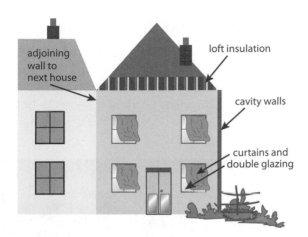

adjoining wall to next house

loft insulation

cavity walls

curtains and double glazing

Note that a well-insulated house will also keep cooler during hot weather.

Payback time is the time it takes for a heat-saving measure to save as much in heating bills as it originally cost to buy.

When considering the effectiveness of saving energy in a home, you should also take account of:

- the thickness of the walls.
- the area and number of windows.
- the fact that a detached house has a greater surface area than a terraced house.

SUMMARY

- **Heat moves through solids by conduction. Metals are good conductors of heat, whilst plastics and wood are poor conductors.**

- **Heat can move through gases and liquids by convection. Hot liquids / gases rise as they become less dense. Cooler liquids / gases sink as they are more dense.**

- **Radiation is the transfer of energy by infrared electromagnetic waves. It can occur in a vacuum.**

- **Houses are insulated to reduce heat loss.**

QUESTIONS

QUICK TEST

1. Name the **three** ways that heat can move.
2. Which type of heat transfer occurs best in solids?
3. Why does hot air rise?
4. What sort of body absorbs and emits a large amount of radiation?
5. Give **three** ways of improving the insulation of a house.

EXAM PRACTICE

1. What happens when infrared radiation comes into contact with:

   a) a dark matt surface? **(1 mark)**

   b) a light shiny surface? **(1 mark)**

2. The table below shows the initial cost and annual saving on energy bills of three different methods of insulation.

Method	Initial Cost (£)	Annual Saving on Energy Bills (£)
Loft Insulation	500	250
Double Glazing	2000	300
Cavity Wall Insulation	5000	500

   a) Which of the above methods reduces heat loss the most in a year? **(1 mark)**

   b) Explain which of the above methods has the shortest payback time. **(2 marks)**

3. Explain how the design features of a home can help to prevent heat loss.

   The quality of written communication will be assessed in your answer to this question.
   (6 marks)

Heat

Trapping Heat Energy

Nearly all of our energy comes from the Sun.

Solar panels use energy from the Sun to heat up water in pipes to use for heating. Solar panels are painted black to increase the absorption of radiation.

Photocells (**solar cells**) convert the Sun's energy directly into electricity.

Some information about photocells is given below:

- Photocells work by absorbing energy that knocks electrons loose from silicon atoms in the crystals.
- Electrons then flow freely to produce direct current.
- The power of photocells depends on their surface area and the light intensity.
- Photocells can operate in remote locations.
- Photocells produce no waste.
- Photocells are low maintenance.
- Photocells do not work in bad weather or at night.

Passive solar heating works because glass allows the Sun's radiation to pass through, but it reflects the **infrared radiation** given off by the heated surfaces inside.

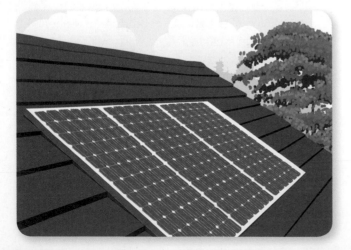

Temperature and Heat Transfer

Temperature is a measurement of hotness (concentration of heat energy) and is measured in degrees **Celsius** (°C). Heat is a measurement of energy and is measured in joules (J). Temperature can be represented by a range of colours in a thermogram, like the one shown here.

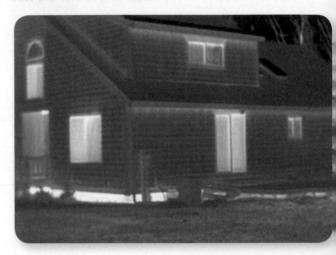

Here are some factors that affect the rate at which heat is transferred:

- If a body is warmer (at a higher temperature) than its surroundings, it will lose heat energy to its surroundings. The greater the temperature difference, the faster the rate at which heat is transferred.
- If a body is cooler (at a lower temperature) than its surroundings, it will gain heat energy from its surroundings. The greater the temperature difference, the faster the rate at which heat is transferred.
- Under similar conditions, different materials transfer heat at different rates. In a cold room, a carpet does not transfer heat very quickly (it is a good thermal insulator). If you walk on the carpet without shoes you will not feel cold because the heat is being transferred away from your warmer feet at a slow rate. However, if you walk on a tiled floor at the same temperature, your feet will feel cold. This is because the tiles transfer heat away from your feet faster (they are good thermal conductors).

The shape and the dimensions of a body affect the rate at which it transfers heat. A body with a larger surface area will lose heat quickly. For example, babies have a large surface area compared with their volume – this is one reason why it is more difficult for babies to keep warm.

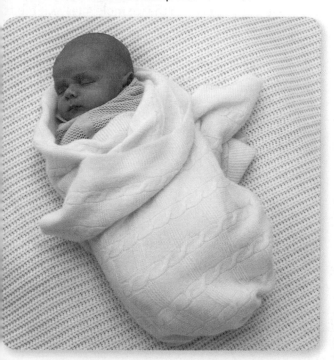

QUESTIONS

QUICK TEST

1. Why are solar panels painted black?

2. What is temperature?

3. What is heat?

4. Why is it difficult for babies to keep warm?

5. Why does a tiled floor feel cold?

EXAM PRACTICE

1. Steph was organising a scientific expedition to the Gobi desert. She was considering taking some photocells to power her laptop.

   a) What are the advantages to Steph of using photocells? **(3 marks)**

   b) Are there any disadvantages to using photocells? **(2 marks)**

2. The diagrams show an experiment with a small solar cell.

A

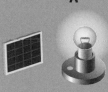

B

   a) Explain why the output of the solar cells would differ in positions A and B. **(2 marks)**

   b) What else could affect the output? **(1 mark)**

Heat Calculations

Specific Heat Capacity

The energy needed to change the temperature of a body depends on:

● its mass
● the material it is made from
● the temperature change required.

The **specific heat capacity** tells us how much energy 1 kg of a material needs to increase its temperature by 1°C. The unit of specific heat capacity is joules per kg per degree.

The energy required to heat a substance, or the heat lost by a substance when cooling, is calculated using the following equation:

$$\text{Energy} = \text{mass} \times \frac{\text{specific heat capacity}}{} \times \frac{\text{temperature change}}{}$$

Example

500 g of water is allowed to cool from 80 °C to 55 °C. How much energy is lost to its surroundings? (specific heat capacity of water is 4200 J/kg/°C)

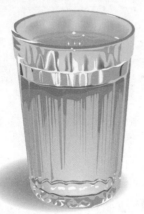

Energy = 0.5 kg × 4200 J/kg/°C × 25 °C
     = **52 500 J**

When heating a substance, some of the energy is lost to the surroundings. Therefore, we calculate the **minimum** amount of energy required.

Specific Latent Heat

If we steadily heat ice at −20 °C its temperature increases steadily until it reaches 0 °C.

The ice continues to absorb energy at the same rate without getting any hotter, using the energy to break down the bonds between the ice molecules as it melts.

As a substance is heated or cooled, a graph can show the change in temperature.

The graph below shows ice as it is heated and melts, and then heated (as water) and evaporates.

The heating takes place at a constant rate, so rate of heat added is proportional to the time.

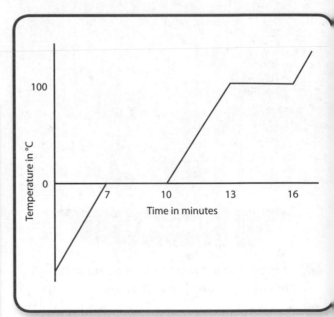

● The horizontal section from 7 to 10 minutes shows that the ice is absorbing heat energy as it changes from ice to water at a constant temperature of 0 °C.
● Between 10 minutes and 13 minutes, the substance is liquid water.
● The horizontal section from 13 minutes to 16 minutes shows the water absorbing heat as it evaporates at 100 °C.

The energy required to melt a substance is the **latent heat**. Liquid requires latent heat to evaporate. Gases lose heat as they condense, and liquids lose heat as they freeze. All changes happen at a constant temperature.

The **specific latent heat** of a substance is the amount of energy required to change the state of 1 kg of that substance at a constant temperature.

We can calculate latent heat using the following equation:

Energy = mass × specific latent heat

SUMMARY

- The energy needed to change the temperature of a body depends on its mass, the material it is made from, and the temperature change required.

- Energy loss or gain can be calculated by:

  Energy = mass × specific heat capacity × temperature change

- The energy required to change the state of a substance can be calculated by:

  Energy = mass × specific latent heat

QUESTIONS

QUICK TEST

1. What is specific heat capacity?

2. At what temperatures does water freeze and melt?

3. What is specific latent heat?

4. Calculate the minimum energy needed to raise the temperature of 2 kg of water by 5 °C.

5. Calculate the energy lost when 1 kg of copper cools by 5 °C (specific heat capacity= 385 J/kg/°C).

EXAM PRACTICE

1. What **three** things does the energy needed to change the temperature of a material depend on?   **(3 marks)**

2. Look at the data in the table opposite.

   a) Which material will require the most energy to raise its temperature by 1 °C? Explain your answer.   **(2 marks)**

   b) Calculate the energy needed to raise the temperature of 2 kg of titanium by 10 °C.   **(1 mark)**

Material	Specific Heat Capacity (J/kg/°C)
Aluminium	880
Titanium	523
Water	4200

3. The specific latent heat of ice is 330 J/g. How much energy is required to melt 30 g of ice?   **(1 mark)**

4. Colin carries out an experiment using 2 kg of paraffin wax. It takes 30 000 J of energy to raise the temperature by 6 °C. Calculate the specific heat capacity of paraffin wax.   **(2 marks)**

Temperature and Pressure

Heat is a measurement of energy and is measured in joules (J). Usually temperature is measured in degrees Celsius (°C).

Water freezes and ice melts at 0 °C and water evaporates and steam condenses at 100 °C.

As particles are heated, the extra energy causes them to move or vibrate faster. As particles lose energy their movement decreases.

At a temperature of –273 °C all particles, regardless of their type, stop moving altogether. This temperature is known as **absolute zero**.

The Celsius temperature scale is based on the freezing point and the boiling point of water.

In the 19th Century, a man called Lord Kelvin designed a new temperature scale based on absolute zero. The increments between each point on the Kelvin temperature scale are the same as the increments on the Celsius scale, but zero Kelvin is equal to –273 °C, i.e. absolute zero.

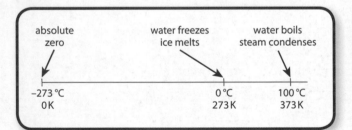

absolute zero	water freezes ice melts	water boils steam condenses
–273 °C 0 K	0 °C 273 K	100 °C 373 K

To change from:

⬤ Kelvin to degrees Celsius, add 273

⬤ degrees Celsius to Kelvin, subtract 273.

The Kelvin temperature of a gas is **directly proportional** to the average kinetic energy of its particles.

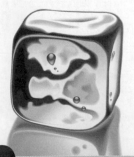

The Gas Laws

Pressure in a gas is caused by particles bombarding the surface of the container they are in. Hotter particles move faster, and bombard the surface more frequently and with greater force.

For a gas in a sealed container (at constant volume), pressure is proportional to temperature in Kelvin. The unit of pressure is **Pascals** (Pa).

$$\frac{P}{T} = \text{constant}$$

P = Pressure T = Temperature in Kelvin

Example

Consider a gas is at a temperature of 15 °C at a pressure of 140 000 Pa. If the gas is heated at constant volume to a temperature of 45 °C, find its new pressure.

15 °C = 288 K and 45 °C = 318 K

At 288 K $\frac{P}{T} = \frac{140\,000\,\text{Pa}}{288\,\text{K}}$

= 486 Pa/K

Pressure at 318 K = 486 Pa/K × 318 K

= **155 000 Pa**

If the gas is not kept at constant volume, the equation below can be used.

$$\frac{P_1 V_1}{T_1} = \frac{P_2 V_2}{T_2}$$

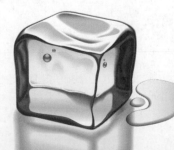

Example

Consider an air bubble underwater at a temperature of 10 °C, a pressure of 200 000 Pa with a volume of 30 cm^3.

Find the new volume of the bubble if it rises to the surface where the temperature is 25 °C and the pressure is 100 000 Pa.

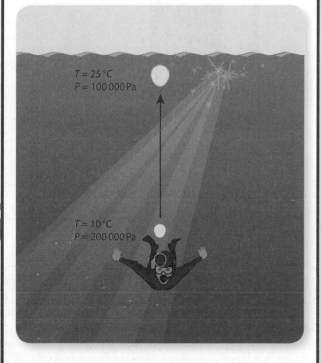

$T = 25$ °C
$P = 100 000$ Pa

$T = 10$ °C
$P = 200 000$ Pa

10 °C = 283 K and 25 °C = 298 K

Since the equation uses ratios, the volume can remain in cm^3.

$$\frac{200\,000\,Pa \times 30\,cm^3}{283\,K} = \frac{100\,000\,Pa \times V}{298\,K}$$

$$21\,201.41 = \frac{(100\,000 \times V)}{298}$$

$$21\,201.41 \times 298 = 100\,000 \times V$$

$$\frac{(21\,210.41 \times 298)}{100\,000} = V$$

$$V = \textbf{63 cm}^3$$

SUMMARY

● **The coldest possible temperature is called absolute zero. Absolute zero is –273 °C or 0 Kelvin.**

● **The pressure of a gas is caused by the particles of the gas hitting the sides of the container they are in.**

● **The higher the temperature, the more kinetic energy the particles have and the higher the pressure.**

● **When gas is in a sealed container of constant volume, the pressure is proportional to the temperature in Kelvin.**

QUESTIONS

QUICK TEST

1. Define temperature.

2. Define heat.

3. What is the name given to the temperature –273 °C?

4. What happens to particles at –273 °C?

EXAM PRACTICE

1. What is 30°C in Kelvin? **(1 mark)**

2. Ewan is an Arctic scuba diver. He notices that the pressure in his air cylinder decreases when he takes it from the heated boat cabin out into the Arctic air. Explain this effect. **(3 marks)**

3. A gas with a fixed volume has a pressure of 230 000 Pa at 50 °C. What will its pressure be at 90 °C? **(3 marks)**

Inside the Atom

Atoms

An atom has a small central **nucleus** composed of **protons** and **neutrons**, surrounded by **electrons**.

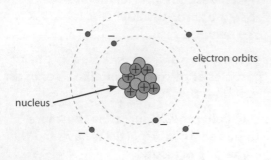

nucleus

electron orbits

Particle	proton	electron	neutron
Charge	+1	−1	none
Mass	1	negligible	1

- The mass (or nucleon) number, A, is the number of nucleons (protons + neutrons).
- The atomic (or proton) number, Z, is the number of protons.

For example, an isotope of radium (Ra) has 226 nucleons, 88 protons and 138 neutrons:

$$^{A}_{Z}X \qquad ^{226}_{88}Ra$$

- Atoms of the same element have the same number of protons.
- Atoms with neutral charge have the same number of electrons as protons.
- An atom may gain or lose electrons to form charged particles called **ions**.
- Atoms with different nucleon numbers have different mass, although they are still the same element. These atoms are called **isotopes**. An isotope of an element has the same number of protons but extra or fewer neutrons.

Radiation

An unstable nucleus may emit radiation. Atoms that give out radiation from their nucleus naturally are said to be **radioactive**.

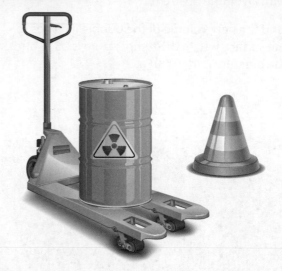

Alpha radiation is a helium nucleus (2 protons and 2 neutrons). It is emitted straight from the nucleus.

For example, radium decays into radon:

$$^{226}_{88}Ra \rightarrow ^{222}_{86}Rn + ^{4}_{2}\alpha$$

Beta radiation is an electron emitted from the nucleus. No electrons exist as electrons in the nucleus.

However, in an unstable nucleus a neutron may spontaneously change into a proton. When it does this, it emits an electron. This is called beta radiation.

For example, iodine decays into xenon.

$$^{128}_{53}I \rightarrow ^{128}_{54}Xe + ^{0}_{-1}\beta$$

Gamma radiation is an electromagnetic wave. It usually follows alpha or beta radiation. X-rays have similar properties to gamma rays, but are emitted from different sources.

Ionisation is the ability of the radiation to cause other particles to gain or to lose electrons.

The table below shows the properties of the three different types of nuclear radiation.

	Alpha	Beta	Gamma
Range in the Air	a few centimetres	about a metre	huge distances
Penetration Power	stopped by a thick sheet of paper or skin	stopped by a few centimetres of aluminium or other metal	lead or thick concrete will reduce its intensity
Ionising Power	strong	weak	very weak
Charge	+2	−1	none

SUMMARY

- **An atom is composed of protons, neutrons and electrons.**

- **A proton and neutron have the same relative mass. An electron has negligible mass.**

- **A proton has a positive charge, an electron has a negative charge, and a neutron has no charge.**

- **Radiation can be divided into alpha, beta and gamma.**

QUESTIONS

QUICK TEST

1. What is the charge on a neutron?

2. What is the range of gamma radiation in air?

3. What is ionisation?

4. What is the ionisation power of alpha radiation?

EXAM PRACTICE

1. An atom of uranium is written as $^{238}_{92}U$.

   a) What is the name given to atoms of the same element with different numbers of neutrons? **(1 mark)**

   b) How many neutrons does each atom of uranium have? **(1 mark)**

   c) An atom of uranium decays by alpha emission. Write an equation for this decay. **(2 marks)**

2. In a laboratory a piece of equipment needs to be shielded from alpha and beta radiation. Explain what type of material should be used. **(3 marks)**

Smaller Particles

If the number of neutrons is plotted against the number of protons for stable isotopes, the curve below is obtained.

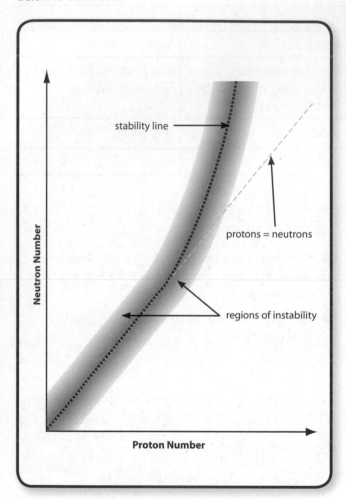

If an isotope does not lie on this curve, it can be identified as unstable and radioactive.

- An isotope above the curve has too many neutrons and will undergo **β⁻ decay**, emitting an electron.
- An isotope below the curve has too few neutrons and will undergo **β⁺ decay**, emitting a positron.
- Nuclei that undergo β⁻ or β⁺ decay often undergo rearrangement, with a loss of energy emitted as **γ radiation**.
- Nuclei with more than 82 protons usually undergo **α decay**.

A **positron** is an electron's **anti-particle**; it is identical to an electron but with positive charge. In an unstable nucleus, a proton may spontaneously change into a neutron plus a positron. The positron is emitted as β⁺ decay.

For example, carbon decays into boron. A particle called a **neutrino** is also produced:

$$^{11}_{6}\text{C} \rightarrow {}^{11}_{5}\text{B} + {}^{0}_{+1}\beta$$

Anti-matter is very similar to ordinary matter, but when matter and anti-matter meet they annihilate each other, releasing energy.

Scientists try to discover more about particles. One way they do this is by accelerating particles close to the speed of light and allowing them to collide.

Fundamental Particles

As far as we know, **fundamental particles** are the smallest particles into which matter can be divided.

There are two groups of fundamental particles: **quarks** and **leptons** (and their anti-particles: anti-quarks and anti-leptons). An electron is a lepton, a positron is an anti-lepton.

There are six 'flavours' of quarks: up, down, strange, charm, bottom and top.

- Protons can be broken into two up quarks and one down quark. The charges combine to give an overall charge of +1.
- Neutrons can be broken into two down quarks and one up quark. The charges combine to give an overall neutral charge.
- β⁻ decay involves the change of a down quark in a neutron to an up quark. The neutron becomes a proton with a charge of +1 plus an electron.
- β⁺ decay involves the change of an up quark in a proton to a down quark. The proton becomes a neutron with no charge plus a positron.

Electron Beams

Thermionic emission is when electrons are 'boiled off' hot metal filaments. The following arrangement produces a beam of electrons equivalent to an electric current.

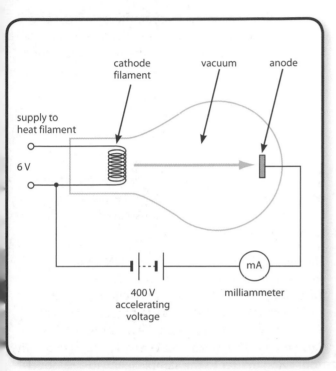

The kinetic energy (KE) of the electrons can be found using this equation:

$$KE = \text{electronic charge} \times \text{accelerating voltage}$$

The principal uses of electron beams are:

- television tubes
- oscilloscopes
- the production of X-rays.

The electrons in these devices are deflected by an electric field created by parallel charged metal plates. The mass of the particle and the strength of the field affect the deflection.

SUMMARY

- Number of neutrons plotted against number of protons gives us a curve we can use to identify unstable and radioactive isotopes.

- Fundamental particles are the smallest particles that matter can be divided into.

- Thermionic emission is when electrons are 'boiled off' hot metal filaments. It can be used in oscilloscopes and to produce X-rays.

QUESTIONS

QUICK TEST

1. What is a positron?

2. Give **two** examples of fundamental particles.

3. What is thermionic emission?

4. State **three** uses of an electron beam.

5. How can electron beams be deflected?

EXAM PRACTICE

1. **a)** Sketch a graph of proton number against neutron number. **(1 mark)**

   b) Show on your graph a possible position of an isotope that:

   i) is stable **(1 mark)**

   ii) will undergo β⁻ decay **(1 mark)**

   iii) will undergo β⁺ decay. **(1 mark)**

Uses of Radiation

Some Uses of Radiation

Radiation can be very useful and has improved the quality of human life in areas such as medicine and industry.

Alpha radiation is used in smoke alarms.

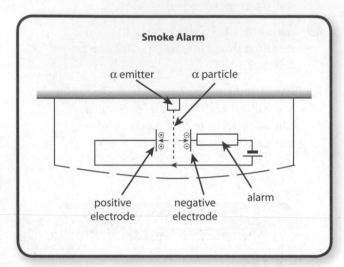

Smoke Alarm

α emitter　　α particle

positive electrode　　negative electrode　　alarm

Beta or gamma radiation can be used as tracers in industry and for diagnostic purposes in hospitals.

- In hospitals, a tracer is swallowed or injected into the body. It is followed on the outside by a radiation detector. This method is used to check a patient's thyroid gland.
- In industry, tracers are used in underground pipes. A gamma source is normally used so it can penetrate to the surface. The source is tracked by a detector above ground. A leak or a blockage is shown by a reduction in activity.
- Gamma radiation is used to treat food so it keeps longer.
- Gamma radiation is used to sterilise equipment.
- Gamma rays are used to treat cancer. A wide beam is focused on the tumour and rotated around the person with the tumour at the centre. This limits the damage to non-cancerous tissue. Radiation with the least penetrating effect possible and the shortest possible half-life also minimises exposure.

Half-Life

The radioactivity (or activity) of an isotope is the number of decays emitted per second. It decreases over time.

The **half-life** of a radioactive sample is defined as the time it takes for the number of undecayed nuclei to halve. It can also be defined as the time it takes for the count rate (activity) to halve. The half-life for any sample is always constant.

The activity of a sample with a half-life of 2 days will be half its original value in 2 days, a quarter in 4 days, and so on.

A tracer used in medicine must have a half-life that isn't too short (so it has time to travel around the body) or too long (so that it doesn't remain in the body for a long period of time).

The half-life can be used to date artefacts in archaeology and rocks. Archaeologists assume that the amount of Carbon-14 has not changed in the air for thousands of years. When an object (e.g. a tree) dies, gaseous exchange with the air stops. The Carbon-14 in the wood decays and the ratio of activity from living matter to the sample leads to a reasonably accurate date. Radioactive dating of rocks depends on the uranium to lead ratio. Scientific conclusions, such as those from radioactive dating, often carry significant uncertainties.

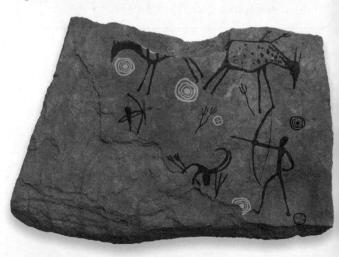

X-Rays

X-rays are used in medicine to view hard tissues in the body such as bones.

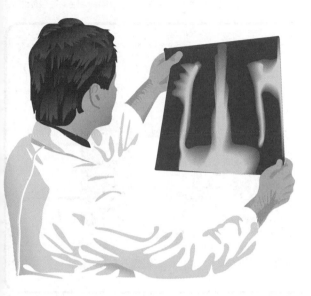

A radiographer is a person who takes X-rays. X-rays and gamma rays have similar wavelengths but are produced in different ways.

Gamma rays are given out from the nuclei of certain radioactive materials. X-rays are made by firing high speed electrons at metal targets, and are easier to control than gamma rays.

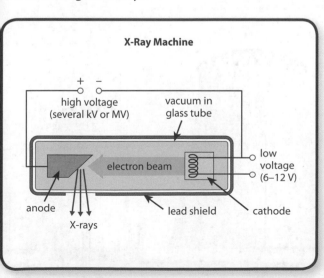

X-Ray Machine

high voltage
(several kV or MV)

vacuum in
glass tube

+ –

electron beam

low
voltage
(6–12 V)

anode

X-rays

lead shield

cathode

SUMMARY

- Radioactive tracers can be used in the human body or industry.

- Gamma rays can be used for sterilisation, preserving food, or treating cancer.

- Radioactive isotopes decay over time. The rate of this decay is the half-life of an isotope.

- X-rays are easier to control than gamma rays.

QUESTIONS

QUICK TEST

1. Suggest a use for alpha radiation.

2. Suggest an industrial use for a tracer.

3. When treating cancer, why is a wide beam of gamma radiation focused on the tumour?

4. What is the difference between X-rays and gamma rays?

5. State an advantage of using X-rays instead of gamma rays.

EXAM PRACTICE

1. Define half-life. **(1 mark)**

2. a) A sample has an activity of 400 counts per second. After 3 days the activity is 200 counts per second. What is the half-life? **(1 mark)**

   b) What will the activity be after 9 days? **(1 mark)**

3. Describe how X-rays are produced in an X-ray tube. **(4 marks)**

Dangers of Radiation

Background Radiation

Background radiation is a low level of radiation that is around us all of the time. It is mainly caused by natural radioactive substances such as rocks, soil, living things and cosmic rays.

Different regions in the UK experience different levels of background radiation. A main cause of this variation is radon gas in the atmosphere.

Humans also contribute to background radiation, for example medical uses, nuclear waste and power stations.

The Earth's atmosphere and magnetic field protect it from radiation from space. The ozone layer protects the Earth from ultraviolet radiation, but pollution from CFCs is depleting the ozone layer.

Risks Associated with Radiation

Radiation can cause cancer or make vital organs stop working.

High levels of radiation pose a greater risk. Over time, scientists have learnt more about the risks associated with radioactive sources.

Here are some general risks associated with radiation:

- Alpha radiation is highly ionising and very dangerous if it is taken into the body. It cannot pass through the skin. However, if it is absorbed in food or by breathing in radioactive gas or dust, the radiation can cause damage deep inside the body.

- Beta and gamma rays can penetrate the skin but most sources of these types of radiation are well shielded, such as in power stations and laboratories.

- Some media reports claim that microwave radiation from mobile phones or masts poses a health risk.

Nuclear Power

Radioactive fuel rods release energy as heat through a process called **nuclear fission**. A nuclear power station uses this heat to drive turbines and generate electricity.

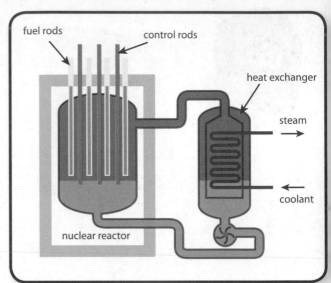

fuel rods | control rods | heat exchanger | steam | coolant | nuclear reactor

Nuclear power stations pose two main risks:

- Accidental emission of radioactive material.
- Waste material disposal.

A radioactive leak could cause damage to humans and wildlife for many years. Radioactive dust can be carried by the wind for thousands of kilometres.

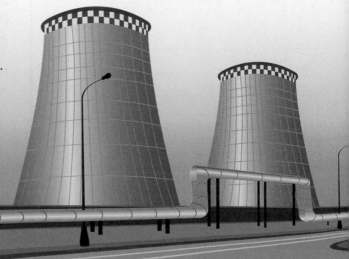

Radioactive Waste

After a few years, the fuel in a reactor must be replaced. The used fuel consists of dangerous radioactive products that need to be stored safely for up to thousands of years. Materials that are near radioactive sources or inside a nuclear reactor absorb extra neutrons, making them radioactive too.

Low-level radioactive waste can be buried in landfill sites. Other waste must be encased in thick glass or concrete and buried. Some types of waste can be reprocessed.

Here are some problems of dealing with radioactive waste:

- It can cause cancer if not disposed of correctly.
- It can remain radioactive for thousands of years.
- Plutonium (waste product from nuclear reactors) can be used to make bombs and could be considered a terrorist risk.
- It must be kept out of groundwater.

Safety in the Laboratory

Radioactive substances must be handled safely in the laboratory:

- Tongs or gloves must be used.
- The exposure time must be minimised.
- Sources should be stored in shielded containers.
- Protective clothing must be worn.

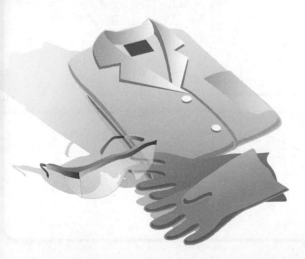

SUMMARY

- There is a low level of background radiation around us at all times. This can come from natural sources or from man-made radiation.
- High levels of radiation are very damaging to human health.
- Nuclear power stations use nuclear fission to produce steam that turns a turbine.

QUESTIONS

QUICK TEST

1. State **three** sources of background radiation.

2. Can gamma radiation penetrate the skin?

3. For how long can nuclear waste remain radioactive?

4. How can nuclear waste be disposed of?

EXAM PRACTICE

1. Local residents often protest when there are plans to build a nuclear power station in their area. What are they likely to be concerned about? **(3 marks)**

2. Why is it more important to shield a beta or gamma source than an alpha source? **(2 marks)**

Radiation and Science

Throughout history, scientific ideas and theories about radiation have been changed and developed as new discoveries are made.

Some theories, such as **Einstein's** theory of relativity, do not originate from experiments. Einstein used his imagination and carried out 'thought' experiments.

Einstein's theory led to predictions which were tested successfully. These tests involved atomic clocks and cosmic rays. The results agreed with the theory and led to more people accepting the ideas.

Without testing new theories, scientists are often reluctant to accept them, especially when they overturn long-established explanations.

Another example of a new theory is '**cold fusion**'. Usually fusion requires extremely high temperatures and densities. Theories such as 'cold fusion' are not accepted until they have been validated by the scientific community.

The Plum Pudding Model

Scientists used to believe that atoms were the smallest particles that existed.

In 1897, **J. J. Thompson** discovered tiny, negatively charged particles, which he named electrons. Thompson found that atoms sometimes give out electrons. Since the overall charge of an atom is neutral, Thompson deduced that an atom might consist of a sphere of positively charged mass with negative electrons inside it.

This model of the atom is known as the 'plum pudding' model since the electrons look a little like plums in a pudding.

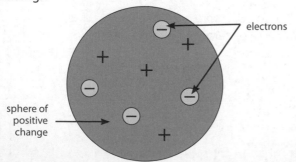

electrons

sphere of positive change

The Nuclear Model

The scientist **Ernest Rutherford** had two assistants, Hans Geiger and Ernest Marsden. In 1911, Rutherford asked them to carry out a new experiment to discover more about atoms.

In the experiment, a thin piece of gold foil was bombarded with alpha particles. Gold foil was chosen because it is very thin. Alpha particles are tiny positive particles emitted by some radioactive substances.

Rutherford found that nearly all of the alpha particles went straight through the gold foil. Very, very few of the alpha particles were deflected by the atoms in the foil.

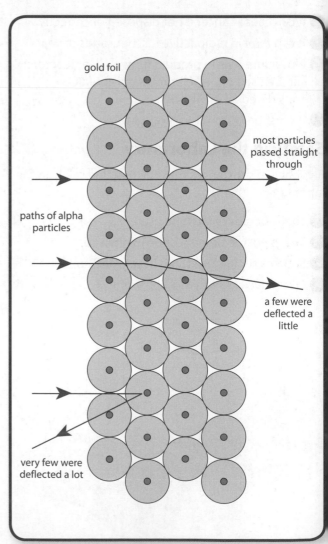

gold foil

most particles passed straight through

paths of alpha particles

a few were deflected a little

very few were deflected a lot

Rutherford concluded that:

- most of an atom is empty space
- most of the mass of an atom is compressed into a tiny volume in the centre called a nucleus
- the nucleus of an atom has an overall positive charge.

Rutherford's new nuclear model of the atom proposed that tiny negatively charged electrons orbited around a dense positive nucleus.

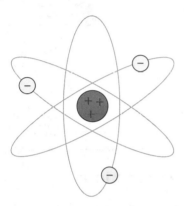

Modern Models

Other scientists have refined Rutherford's model with the discovery of neutrons and energy levels for the electrons.

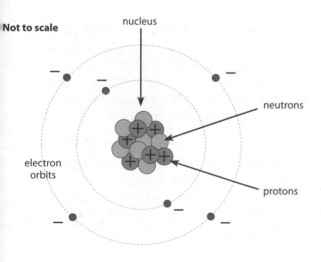

Scientists recently discovered that electrons can behave like clouds of charge, or even waves.

Today, scientists use a mathematical model of an atom using wave mechanics.

SUMMARY

- Scientists develop theories that lead to predictions, which can then be tested.
- The original theory of atomic structure was known as the 'plum pudding' model.
- The plum pudding model was disproved by Ernest Rutherford's experiments.
- Using the data from his experiments, Rutherford developed the nuclear model of the atom, which we use today.

QUESTIONS

QUICK TEST

1. How does testing a model change the way scientists think about it?

2. Give an example of a recent model that needed testing.

3. What particle did Thompson discover?

4. Why is Thompson's model called the 'plum pudding'?

5. What extra information do we know about electrons today?

EXAM PRACTICE

1. A group of scientists claim to have successfully carried out an experiment that proves 'cold fusion'. Why is it important that the experimental method and any data from this experiment are shared with the scientific community? **(3 marks)**

2. Describe how Rutherford's gold foil experiment showed the following:

   a) Most of an atom is empty space. **(2 marks)**

   b) The nucleus of an atom has a positive charge. **(2 marks)**

Nuclear Power

Nuclear Fission

Einstein suggested the possibility of releasing enormous amounts of energy trapped in an atom. **Fission** is the **splitting** of an atom into two lighter nuclei.

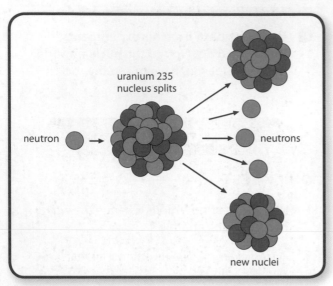

uranium 235 nucleus splits

neutron

neutrons

new nuclei

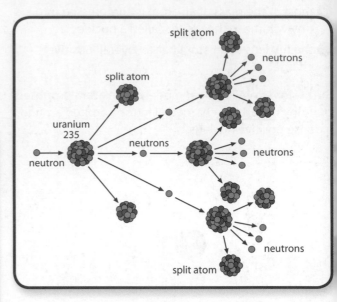

split atom

neutrons

split atom

uranium 235

neutrons

neutrons

neutron

neutrons

split atom

The process:

1. The atom (usually uranium 235) is bombarded with a neutron that is initially absorbed.

2. This makes the nucleus highly unstable.

3. The nucleus splits into two lighter nuclei (daughter nuclei) and releases two or three neutrons.

4. The neutrons bombard other nuclei, causing further splitting.

5. Energy is released rapidly.

This process is known as a **chain reaction**. If the chain reaction is **uncontrolled**, the thermal energy is released extremely rapidly, resulting in an explosion or nuclear bomb.

Nuclear Power Stations

In a nuclear reactor, fission is controlled:

- A **moderator** such as graphite or water slows down the neutrons.

- **Control rods** (that can be raised or lowered) absorb some neutrons but leave enough to keep the reaction going.

A **thermal neutron** has a high kinetic energy and a speed of about 2.2 km/s. If a neutron experiences a number of collisions, it will reach this energy level. Most fission reactors use a moderator to slow down these neutrons so that they interact more easily. Fast breeder reactors use fast neutrons directly.

Radioactive fuel rods such as uranium 235 or plutonium 239 release energy as heat through nuclear fission. In the pressurised reactor on the following page, the hot water is used to produce steam. Steam turns a turbine that drives a generator to produce electricity.

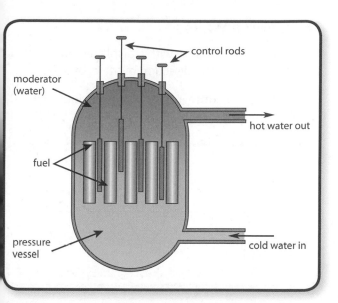

Here are some of the advantages of nuclear power:

- It does not contribute to global warming.
- Small amounts of fuel give large amounts of energy (about a million times more than that from burning).

Here are some disadvantages of nuclear power:

- It has high maintenance costs.
- It has high decommissioning (closing down) costs.
- There is a risk of accidental emission of radioactive material.
- It creates radioactive waste, which can remain dangerously radioactive for thousands of years.

Nuclear Fusion

Nuclear **fusion** is the joining of two atomic nuclei to form a larger one. It is the energy source for stars. It is currently an impractical source of energy due to the extremely high temperatures and densities it requires.

SUMMARY

- Nuclear fission is the splitting of an atom into two lighter nuclei.
- In a nuclear reactor, fission is controlled by a moderator and control rods.
- Radioactive waste can remain dangerously radioactive for thousands of years.
- Nuclear fusion is the joining of two atomic nuclei to form a larger one.

QUESTIONS

QUICK TEST

1. In a chain reaction, a particle is split. What are the products?
2. What does the name 'daughter nuclei' refer to?
3. What is nuclear fusion?

EXAM PRACTICE

1. Why can nuclear fission using uranium 235 as a fuel be described as a chain reaction?
   (3 marks)

2. Why can't nuclear fusion be used to produce power efficiently at the moment? **(2 marks)**

3. Explain how radiation is used to produce electricity.

   The quality of written communication will be assessed in your answer to this question.
   (6 marks)

Waves

Waves transmit energy from one place to another, either through space or through a material.

The wave equation states that for any wave:

> Speed = frequency × wavelength

- **Frequency** is the number of waves passing a point per second and is measured in Hertz (Hz).
- **Wavelength** is the distance between any point on a wave and the same point on the next wave.
- **Amplitude** is the maximum displacement of the waves from rest position.
- **Time period** (T) is the total time taken for a single wave to pass a point. It can be calculated using the equation:

$$T = \frac{1}{frequency}$$

There are two types of wave: **transverse** and **longitudinal**.

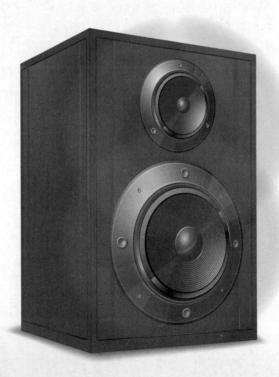

Transverse Waves

Transverse waves vibrate with a displacement **perpendicular** to the direction of travel of the wave.

Examples are electromagnetic waves (including light) and water waves.

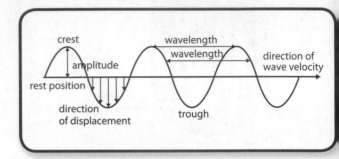

Longitudinal Waves

Longitudinal waves vibrate with a displacement **parallel** to the direction of travel of the wave.

An example are sound waves.

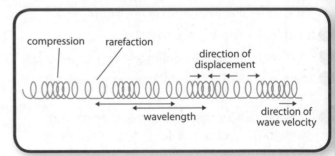

When sound travels through air, the particles vibrate backwards and forwards, parallel to the direction of the wave.

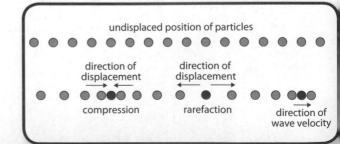

Seismic Waves

Seismic waves are produced by earthquakes as shock waves, and can be detected by seismometers.

- **P-waves** (primary waves) travel through solid and liquid rock. They are longitudinal.

- **S-waves** (secondary waves) travel through solid rock only. They travel slower than P-waves. They are transverse.

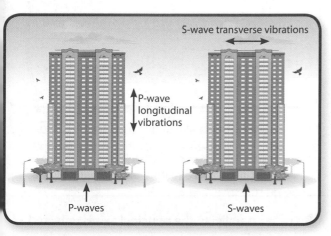

Data from seismic waves can be used to draw conclusions about the types of materials that are found inside the Earth. The outer core stops the S-waves because it is liquid. The waves are also refracted within the mantle due to the different densities of the rock.

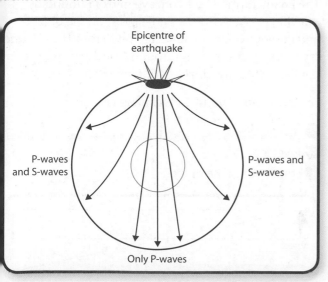

SUMMARY

- **Wave speed = frequency × wavelength**
- **Waves can be either transverse or longitudinal.**
- **There are two types of seismic waves produced by earthquakes: P-waves and S-waves.**
- **P-waves travel through solid and liquid rock; S-waves travel through solid rock only.**

QUESTIONS

QUICK TEST

1. Define wavelength.

2. Define amplitude.

3. What is the time period of a wave?

4. Which type of wave has compressions and rarefactions?

5. Which type of wave has peaks and troughs?

EXAM PRACTICE

1. Mike counts the number of waves that pass a point in 50 seconds. He counts 200 waves. Calculate the frequency of the wave. **(1 mark)**

2. The speed of sound in air is 330 m/s. Calculate the wavelength of a sound wave that has a frequency of 250 Hz. **(1 mark)**

3. What can we deduce about the Earth's core from the way P-waves and S-waves travel after an earthquake?

   The quality of written communication will be assessed in your answer to this question.

   (6 marks)

Reflection

Plane Mirrors

When light is **reflected** by a plane (straight) mirror, the angle of **incidence** is equal to the angle of **reflection**.

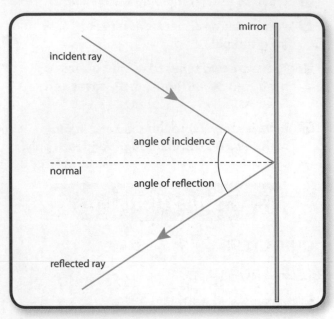

The **normal** is a constructed line perpendicular to any reflecting surface at the point where the incident ray hits the surface.

The nature of an image is defined by:

● whether it is **upright** or **inverted**
● its **size** relative to the object
● whether it is **real** or **virtual**. A real image can be focused on a screen. A virtual image cannot – you have to look into the mirror to see it.

An image in a plane mirror is:

● upright
● virtual
● the same size as the object.

Concave Mirrors

A curved mirror can be **concave** or **convex**. A concave mirror converges parallel rays so that they all pass through the **principal focus**, F.

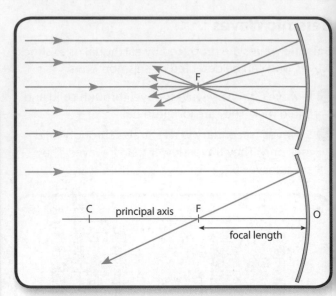

The **focal length** is half the distance to the radius of curvature, C. Both F and C lie on the **principal axis**.

Rays of light reflected at a convex mirror obey the following rules:

● Any ray parallel to the principal axis is reflected through F.
● Any ray passing through F is reflected back parallel to the principal axis.
● Any ray passing through C is reflected back (on itself) through C.

The image formed by a concave mirror is found by drawing two rays from a single point on the object and finding where the reflected rays cross. Usually one ray is drawn that passes through C and another that is parallel to the principal axis and reflected through F.

For an object beyond C, the image is:

● real
● inverted
● smaller than the object.

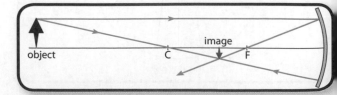

For an object at C, the image is:

- real
- inverted
- the same size as the object.

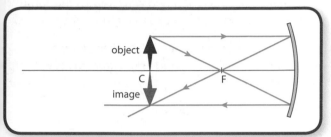

For an object between C and F, the image is:

- real
- inverted
- larger than the object.

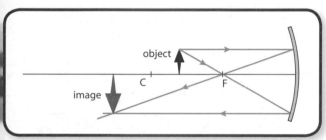

For an object closer than F, the image is:

- virtual
- upright
- magnified.

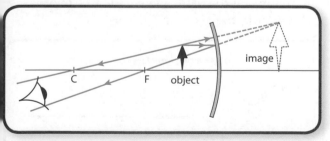

Concave shapes are used for:

- shaving and make-up mirrors
- satellite dishes – microwave signals are brought to a focus
- reflectors in torches and car headlights that form a parallel beam from a light placed at their focal point.

Convex Mirrors

Convex or diverging mirrors form an upright, virtual image that is smaller than the object. Convex mirrors give a wider angle of view and are sometimes used as driving mirrors.

SUMMARY

- When light is reflected by a plane mirror, the angle of incidence is equal to the angle of reflection.

- The focal length (F) of a concave mirror is half the distance to the radius of the curvature (C). An object's position in relation to F and C determines the properties of the image: upright or inverted, size and whether it is real or virtual.

- Convex mirrors form an upright, virtual image that is smaller than the object.

QUESTIONS

QUICK TEST

1. What law governs reflection in a plane mirror?
2. State **three** properties of an image in a plane mirror.
3. What is a normal?

EXAM PRACTICE

1. Explain how a real image differs from a virtual image. **(3 marks)**

2. Explain how the following images could be produced using a concave mirror:

   a) A real, inverted image that is larger than the object. **(1 mark)**

   b) A virtual, upright, magnified image. **(1 mark)**

   c) A real, inverted image that is smaller than the object. **(1 mark)**

Wave Behaviour 1

Diffraction

Diffraction is the spreading out of waves when they pass through a gap. The waves spread out in all directions with **circular wavefronts**. Wavefronts are lines drawn one wavelength apart, perpendicular to the direction of the waves. Diffraction does not affect the wavelength.

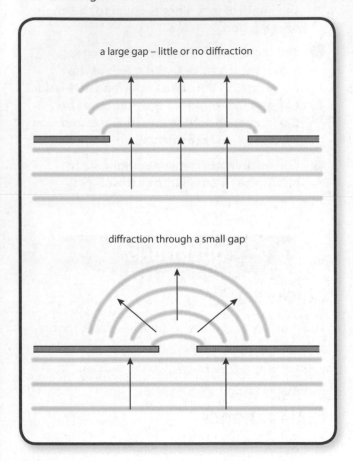

a large gap – little or no diffraction

diffraction through a small gap

Diffraction only happens if the size of the gap is comparable to the wavelength of the wave. The wavelength of visible light is very small (less than 10^{-6} m), which is why visible light does not diffract when it passes through doorways.

Long-wave radio waves have wavelengths much larger, and will diffract around a hill or over the horizon.

Microwave signals to satellites are sent as a thin beam because they will only diffract a small amount due to their short wavelength.

Interference

Interference occurs when two waves (with the same source or the same or a very similar frequency) meet.

Interference effects can be observed in all types of waves including light, sound and water waves in a ripple tank.

There are two types of interference:

● Constructive
● Destructive

In **constructive interference**, the waves must be in **phase** (i.e. arriving 'in step'). This means the path difference for the two waves is an even number of half wavelengths.

The waves combine to give a wave of greater amplitude (hence **constructive** interference as the wave is being 'built up').

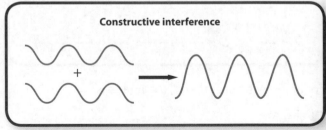

Constructive interference

In **destructive interference**, the waves are not in phase (i.e. they are arriving 'out of step') so they cancel out. This means the path difference for the two waves is an **odd number**.

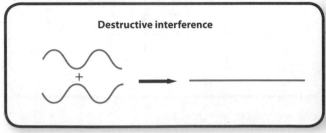

Destructive interference

Coherent wave sources:

● have the same frequency
● are in phase
● have the same amplitude.

Polarisation

Polarisation filters out transverse waves, leaving only those that oscillate in a single plane.

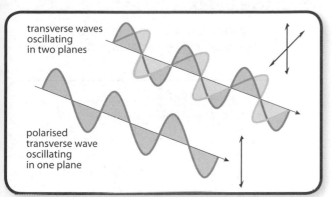

transverse waves oscillating in two planes

polarised transverse wave oscillating in one plane

Unpolarised transverse waves such as electromagnetic waves oscillate in all planes, although they can be thought of as oscillating in two planes: horizontally and vertically. After waves have been polarised, all waves have been filtered out except those oscillating in one plane.

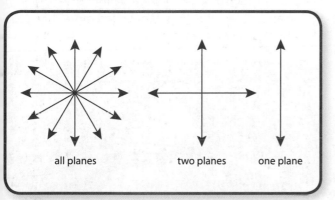

all planes   two planes   one plane

Polaroid sunglasses filter out light in this way. Longitudinal waves cannot be polarised.

SUMMARY

- **Diffraction is the spreading out of waves when they pass through a gap.**

- **When two waves overlap, they produce a pattern of reinforcement and cancellation. This is known as interference.**

- **Polarisation filters transverse waves, leaving only those that oscillate in a single plane.**

QUESTIONS

QUICK TEST

1. What is a wavefront?

2. What is constructive interference?

3. For constructive interference, what is the path difference?

4. Can longitudinal waves be polarised?

5. State a use of polarisation.

EXAM PRACTICE

1. What is diffraction? **(1 mark)**

2. What happens to the wavelength during diffraction? **(1 mark)**

3. **a)** Complete the diagram below to show the diffraction patterns for each gap. **(2 marks)**

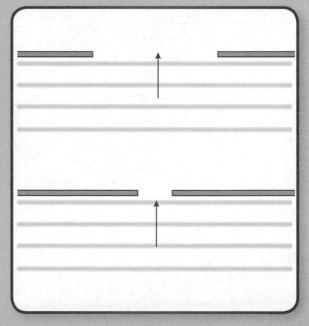

b) Explain why the two patterns are different. **(2 marks)**

Wave Behaviour 2

Refraction

Refraction is when a wave changes direction as it travels from one medium to another. This is a result of a change of speed as the wave enters a new material. For example, water waves slow down when the water depth decreases.

Light slows down when it enters water or glass from air, and speeds up when it leaves. Refraction causes swimming pools to look shallower than they really are. This is known as real and apparent depth because the apparent depth is less than the real depth.

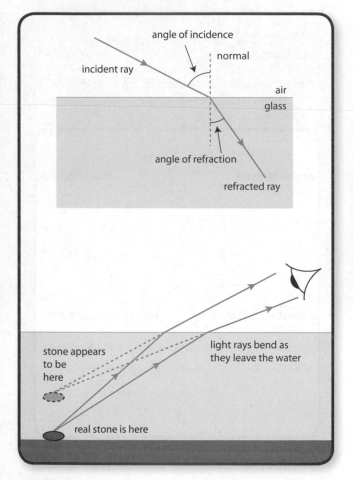

When a light ray slows down, it bends towards the normal, and the angle of refraction is less than the angle of incidence. If it speeds up, it bends away from the normal. If a wave enters a new medium at a right angle, no bending occurs.

Refractive Index

The **refractive index**, n, is constant for any medium. It allows us to calculate the angles of incidence and refraction.

$$n = \frac{\text{speed of light in vacuum}}{\text{speed of light in medium}}$$

$$n = \frac{\sin i}{\sin r}$$

where i is the angle of incidence and r is the angle of refraction.

Dispersion

When a narrow beam of white light passes through a prism, it separates into a spectrum of colour due to refraction. White light is made of all of the colours of the colour spectrum: red, orange, yellow, green, blue, indigo and violet. Blue light is deviated more than red. This effect is called **dispersion**.

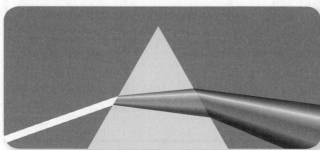

Total Internal Reflection

Visible light rays or infrared can be reflected along the inside of an optical fibre if the **incident angle** is greater than or equal to the **critical angle**. This effect is called **total internal reflection**.

The critical angle depends on the refractive index of the medium inside the optical fibre compared to the medium outside (usually air).

$$\sin c = \frac{n_{\text{outside}}}{n_{\text{inside}}}$$

The higher the refractive index for a material, the lower its critical angle.

Different media have different critical angles. For some types of glass, *c* is equal to about 41°; for acrylic it is 42°.

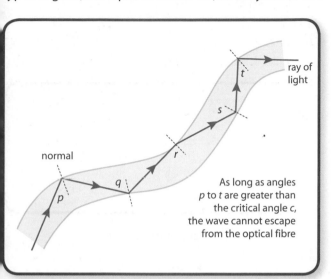

normal

p

q

r

s

t

ray of light

As long as angles *p* to *t* are greater than the critical angle *c*, the wave cannot escape from the optical fibre

⬤ Optical fibres are used in endoscopes – small cameras used to see inside the body.

⬤ Optical fibres can be flexible.

⬤ Optical fibres can transmit data at high speeds.

⬤ The pulses of light are digital signals.

⬤ Many digital pulses can be sent on the same data line (multiplexing), allowing more information to be transmitted.

⬤ Digital signals are clearer; they create less interference.

SUMMARY

⬤ **Refraction is when a wave changes direction as it travels from one medium to another.**

⬤ **When a narrow beam of white light passes through a prism it separates into a spectrum. This is known as dispersion.**

⬤ **Total internal reflection can be used to transmit information along an optical fibre.**

QUESTIONS

QUICK TEST

1. What is refraction?

2. Give an example of when light speeds up.

3. Why does a swimming pool seem shallower than it really is?

4. Define dispersion.

5. What is multiplexing?

EXAM PRACTICE

1. The diagram shows a ray of light entering an optical fibre and reflecting off the inside surface.

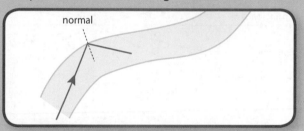

normal

a) What is this effect called? **(1 mark)**

b) Label the angle that must be greater than the critical angle for this to occur. **(1 mark)**

c) Continue the path of the ray as it reflects along the inside of the glass fibre. **(1 mark)**

2. Look at this table showing the refractive index of different wavelengths of light.

Colour of Light	Wavelength in m	Refractive Index
Blue	4.30×10^{-7}	1.53
Red	7.04×10^{-7}	1.51

a) Use the information in the table to explain why the light disperses as it passes through the prism. **(3 marks)**

b) Which colour, red or blue, is slowed down most as it enters the prism? Explain your answer. **(2 marks)**

Lenses

Lenses refract light that passes through them.

The images they form are similar to those formed by curved mirrors. A real image can be focused on a screen. Cameras and projectors form real images.

A **convex** or converging lens forms different images, depending on the position of the object. The position of the image is found by drawing two rays from the object and finding the position where they cross.

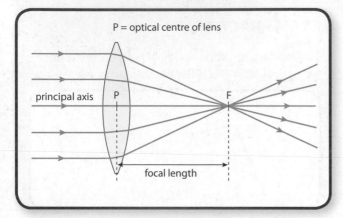

P = optical centre of lens

principal axis   P   F

focal length

Refracted rays obey the following rules:
- Any ray passing through the **optical centre** of the lens, P, is undeflected.
- Any ray parallel to the **principal axis** is refracted through the **focal point**, F.
- Any ray passing through the focal point, F, is refracted parallel to the principal axis.

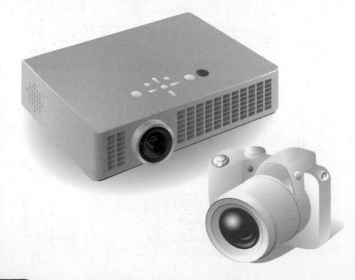

An image formed by an object beyond 2F (2 times focal length) is:
- real
- inverted
- smaller than the object.

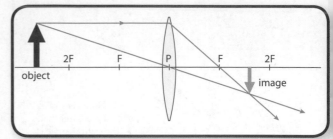

An image formed by an object at 2F is:
- real
- inverted
- the same size as the object.

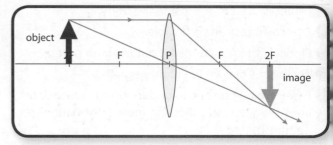

An image formed by an object between F and 2F is:
- real
- inverted
- larger than the object.

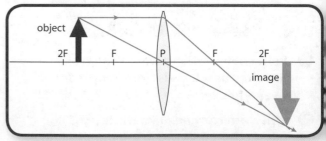

An image formed by an object that is closer than F is:
- virtual
- upright
- magnified.

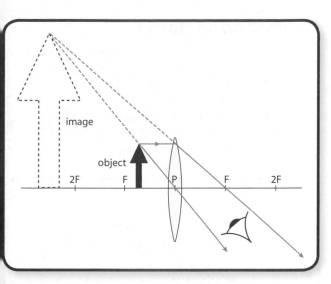

A fatter lens made of the same material as a thinner lens has a shorter focal length.

Convex lenses are used:
- to focus an image on a film in a camera
- in magnifying glasses
- in projectors.

A **concave** or diverging lens forms an upright, virtual image of any object. The image is always closer to the lens than the object and smaller.

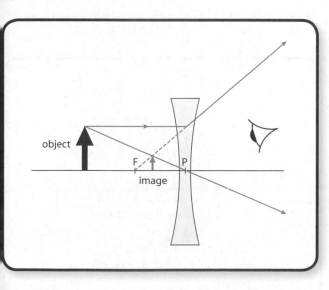

The dashed ray is a virtual ray drawn back to the focal point in order to find the position of the image.

Magnification

A ray diagram can be carefully constructed to scale in order to find the magnification of the image. The magnification of an image formed by a curved mirror or a lens can be found using the following equation:

$$\text{Magnification} = \frac{\text{image height}}{\text{object height}}$$

SUMMARY

- **A convex lens forms different images depending on the position of the object relative to the focal point.**

- **A concave lens forms an upright, virtual image that is smaller than the object.**

- **$\text{Magnification} = \dfrac{\text{image height}}{\text{object height}}$**

QUESTIONS

QUICK TEST

1. State **three** properties of an image formed by a convex lens if the object is placed at 2F.

2. Give **two** properties of an image formed by a concave lens.

EXAM PRACTICE

1. Give **three** uses of convex lenses. **(3 marks)**

2. Kat was examining a spider using a magnifying hand lens. The spider was 0.5 cm long but the image produced was 4 cm long. Calculate the magnification of the hand lens. **(1 mark)**

3. A 26 m image is produced using a magnification of 78 times. Calculate the size of the original object. **(2 marks)**

The Eye

Structure of the Eye

The structure of the human eye is shown below.

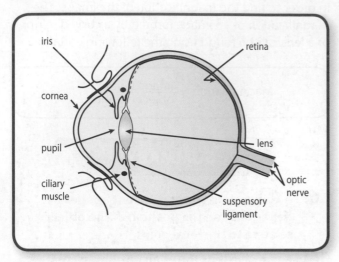

Light enters the eye through the transparent **cornea** which refracts the light.

The light passes through the gap in the **iris** known as the **pupil**. The iris can change the size of the pupil to increase or decrease the amount of light entering the eye.

The lens further refracts the light so that it is focused on the retina. The retina detects the light and sends signals down the **optic nerve**, which are interpreted by the brain.

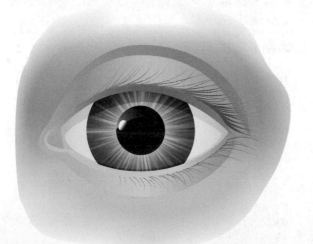

Focusing on an Object

The eye is able to focus on an object between the near point and the far point. The near point of the human eye is 25 cm and the far point is infinity.

In order to focus on a close-up object, the **ciliary muscles** contract and the lens becomes fatter. This causes greater refraction of the light.

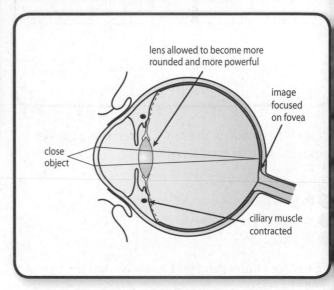

In order to focus on a distant object, the ciliary muscles relax and the lens becomes thinner. This causes a lesser refraction of the light.

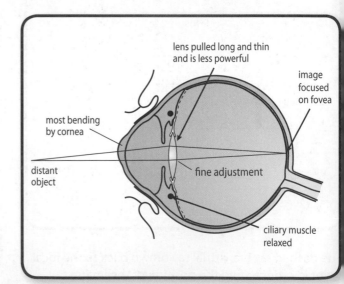

Eye Defects

Two common sight problems are short-sightedness and long-sightedness.

Short-sightedness can be caused by the eyeball being too long or the lens being unable to focus. People who are short-sighted are unable to focus on distant objects.

Long-sightedness can be caused by the eyeball being too short or the lens being unable to focus. People who are long-sighted are unable to focus on near objects.

Both long-sightedness and short-sightedness can be treated in a number of ways:

- Glasses and contact lenses – the lenses of glasses and contact lenses refract the light before it enters the eye. This causes the light to be focused on the retina.
- Laser surgery – a laser is used to reshape the cornea. This causes the light entering the eye to refract differently, focusing the light on the retina.

Cameras

A camera works in a similar way to an eye. The lens on the camera focuses the light on the photographic film or CCD (Charge Coupled Device) in a digital camera.

SUMMARY

- The human eye uses the cornea and lens to focus light on the retina.
- The lens changes shape in order to focus on near or distant objects.
- Long-sightedness and short-sightedness can be corrected using glasses, contact lenses or laser surgery.
- A camera works in a similar way to the eye.

QUESTIONS

QUICK TEST

1. Draw a fully labelled diagram of the human eye.

2. What are the different causes of short- and long-sightedness?

3. In what ways is a camera similar to an eye?

EXAM PRACTICE

1. Explain how the structure of the eye allows it to focus on:

   a) near objects **(3 marks)**

   b) far objects **(3 marks)**

2. The diagram below shows the eye of a person who is long-sighted.

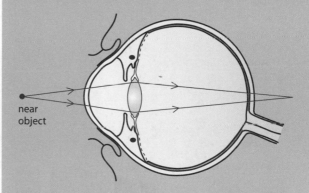

near object

   a) Using the diagram, explain the problems this person experiences with their vision. **(2 marks)**

   b) What could be done to correct these problems? Explain your answer. **(4 marks)**

The Electromagnetic Spectrum

Electromagnetic Radiation

There are many types of **electromagnetic radiation**, including visible light. Different colours of visible light have different **frequencies** and **wavelengths**. Other electromagnetic waves have a wider range of frequencies and wavelengths outside the range of detection of human eyes; they are invisible. All electromagnetic waves travel at the same speed through a vacuum (or air) – the speed of light (300×10^6 m/s).

The Electromagnetic Spectrum

The **electromagnetic spectrum** is continuous, but waves within it are grouped into types as shown below.

Different wavelengths of electromagnetic waves are reflected, refracted, absorbed or transmitted differently by different substances and types of surfaces.

Excessive exposure to **electromagnetic** waves can be detrimental. Higher-frequency radiation causes greater risk.

- **Infrared waves** are given off by heaters; too much can cause skin burns. Particles at the surface absorb infrared and the heat is transferred to the centre by convection or conduction. Infrared sensors are used in remote controls, burglar alarms and short-distance computer data links.

- **Ultraviolet light** is emitted naturally by the Sun. Overexposure damages skin and eyes, and causes cancer. High factor sunblock reduces the risks.

- **Microwaves** are absorbed by particles on the outside layers of food to a depth of about 1 cm, increasing the kinetic energy of the particles. The heat is transferred to the centre by conduction or convection. Microwaves are reflected by metal, but can go through glass and plastics. Microwaves of high frequency and energy can cause burns when absorbed by body tissue.

- **X-rays** and **gamma rays** cause mutation or destruction of cells in the body.

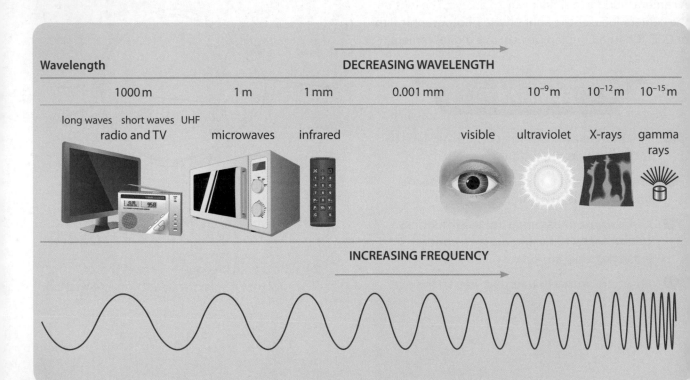

Absorption and Reflection

Different wavelengths of electromagnetic radiation have different effects on living cells. Some pass through, and some are absorbed and produce heat or an alternating current of the same frequency of the radiation. Some cause cancerous changes and some may kill the cells. These effects depend on the type of radiation and the size of the dose.

Here are some applications of scanning by **absorption**:

- Microwaves are used to monitor rain
- X-rays are used to see bone fractures
- Ultraviolet light is used to detect forged bank notes.

Here are some applications of scanning by **reflection**:

- Ultrasound is used to scan a foetus during pregnancy. The distance to the reflecting surface is calculated using:

  $$\text{Speed} = \frac{\text{distance}}{\text{time}}$$

- Optical waves are used for iris recognition.

Radio frequencies below 30 MHz are reflected by the ionosphere. Above 30 GHz, rain, dust and other atmospheric effects reduce the strength of the signal due to absorption and scattering.

Infrared uses scanning by **emission** to monitor temperature.

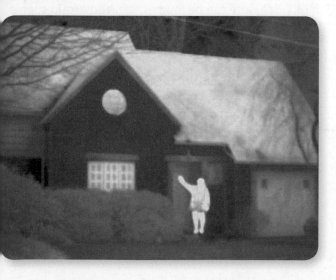

SUMMARY

- **Different colours of visible light have different frequencies and wavelengths.**

- **There are many types of electromagnetic radiation. In order of decreasing wavelength they are: radio and TV waves, microwaves, infrared, visible light, ultraviolet light, X-rays and gamma rays.**

- **Microwaves, X-rays and ultraviolet light are used to scan by absorption.**

- **Ultrasound and visible light are used to scan by reflection.**

QUESTIONS

QUICK TEST

1. Some electromagnetic radiation passes straight through cells, while some causes damage. What **two** properties of the radiation affect what happens?

2. Give another possible effect of radiation on living cells.

3. State **one** application of scanning by absorption.

4. State **one** application of scanning by reflection.

5. State **one** application of scanning by emission.

EXAM PRACTICE

1. What **three** types of radiation can increase the risk of developing cancer? **(3 marks)**

2. A submarine sends down an ultrasound pulse. Ultrasound travels at 1400 m/s. The pulse takes 4 seconds to return to the submarine. How deep is that part of the ocean? **(2 marks)**

3. Why is it not true to say that microwaves cook food from the inside out? **(3 marks)**

Sound

Sounds are mechanical vibrations that can be detected by the human ear. The human ear can detect mechanical vibrations if they are in the frequency range of 20–20 000 Hz.

Sound travels as a wave, usually through air, and is a **longitudinal** wave. Sound waves can be **reflected** and **refracted**.

When sound travels through air, the particles vibrate backwards and forwards, parallel to the direction of the wave.

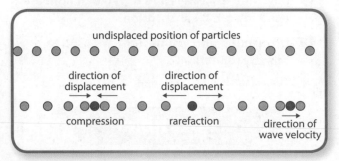

The longitudinal vibrations can be displayed by an oscilloscope using a microphone. The oscilloscope translates the vibrations into an image of a transverse wave. The **amplitude**, the **wavelength** and the **frequency** of the wave can be observed on the trace.

These two waveforms represent sound of different wavelengths and frequencies. The waveform with a high frequency has a shorter wavelength, and the waveform with a low frequency has a longer wavelength.

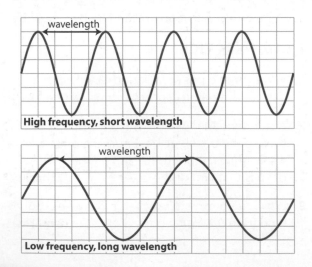

High frequency, short wavelength

Low frequency, long wavelength

Pitch and Volume

The **pitch** (note) of a sound wave depends on the frequency. A high-frequency sound wave has a high pitch (note) and a low-frequency sound wave has a low pitch.

The amplitude of a sound wave determines the **volume** or loudness of the note. A wave with a small amplitude has a soft or quiet note and a wave with a large amplitude is loud.

The two waveforms below represent sound waves of identical frequencies and wavelengths but different amplitudes.

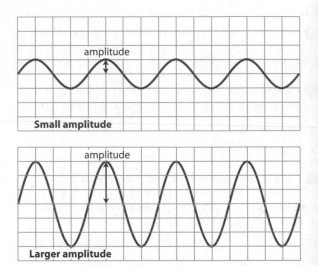

Small amplitude

Larger amplitude

Frequency and amplitude are independent. Therefore, pitch and volume are independent. This means that a high pitch note can be loud or soft, and a loud sound can have a high pitch or a low pitch.

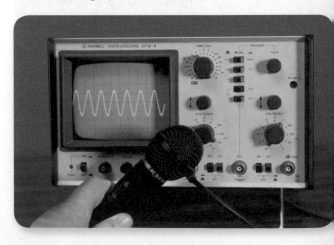

Ultrasound

Ultrasound waves have higher frequency than the upper threshold of human hearing. That means that the frequency of ultrasound is above 20 000 Hz.

Ultrasound waves are partially reflected when they meet a boundary between two different media. The time taken for reflections to reach a detector is a measure of how far away the boundary is.

Ultrasound is used:

- to look inside people (body scans); it reflects at layer boundaries
- for pre-natal scanning
- to break down kidney and other stones
- to measure the speed of blood flow
- for cleaning and control quality in industry.

Ultrasound has advantages over X-rays in that it:

- can produce images of soft tissues
- does not damage living cells.

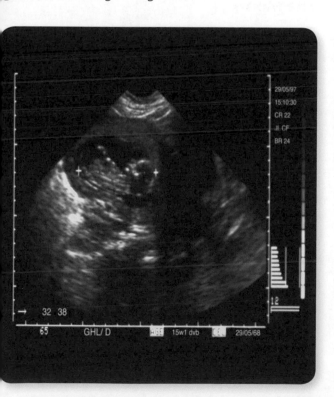

SUMMARY

- Sound waves are longitudinal waves with a frequency range of 20–20 000 Hz.

- The pitch of a sound wave depends on its frequency whilst its volume depends on its amplitude. These are independent of each other.

- Ultrasound has a frequency above 20 000 Hz. It is partially reflected by boundaries between different media so can be used in scanning.

QUESTIONS

QUICK TEST

1. What name is given to sound waves of frequency above the threshold of human hearing?

2. What effect does the amplitude of a sound wave have on the sound it produces?

3. What effect does the frequency of a sound wave have on the sound it produces?

EXAM PRACTICE

1. a) Why is sound described as a longitudinal wave? **(2 marks)**

   b) How can sound be visualised as a transverse wave? **(2 marks)**

2. State two advantages of ultrasound compared to X-rays. **(2 marks)**

3. Explain why frequency and amplitude are said to be independent of each other. **(3 marks)**

Beyond our Planet

The Universe

The **universe** consists of:

- stars and planets
- comets and meteorites
- black holes
- large groups of stars called galaxies.

Our **galaxy** is called the **Milky Way** and consists of billions of stars. In our **solar system**, the Earth is one of many planets orbiting our star (the Sun) with different radiuses and time periods. Gravity provides the centripetal force for orbital motion.

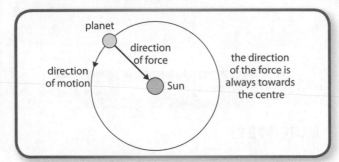

The Earth has an orbit of 365 days. Every 24 hours, it rotates on its axis creating day and night. The existence of life on our planet is determined by the position of our planet within our solar system and the position of our star, the Sun, in its life cycle.

Early Ideas

Thousands of years ago scientists observing our solar system developed the Ptolemaic or **geocentric model**. This model stated that:

- The Earth was the centre of the universe.
- The planets and stars revolved around the Earth.

This model was based on the scientists' observations of the night sky.

In the 16th century, **Copernicus** put forward a different model. This was called the **heliocentric model**.

This model stated that:

- The Sun was the centre of the universe.
- The planets and stars revolved around the Sun.

In the early 17th century, **Galileo** invented the first telescope. This allowed him to study the movement of planets in much more detail. His telescope used an objective lens to produce an image that was then magnified by an eye piece. His observations of Venus proved that the geocentric model could not be correct.

Further work over the next 200 years proved both the Ptolemaic and Copernican models to be incorrect and gave us our modern understanding of the solar system.

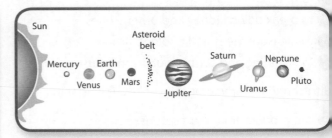

The Moon

The **moon** orbits Earth. The moon may be the remains of a planet that collided with the Earth. When two planets collide, their iron cores can merge to form a larger planet, and the less-dense material orbits as a moon.

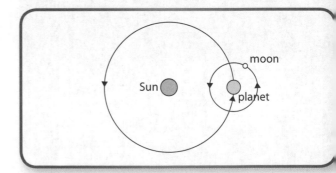

Comets

Comets orbit the Sun with highly elliptical orbits. They are made from ice and dust from far beyond the planets. A comet has least speed when furthest from the Sun, when the gravitational pull is the weakest.

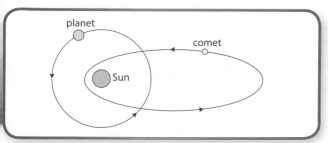

planet

comet

Sun

Asteroids

Asteroids are lumps of rock that orbit the Sun. There are thousands of them, which were left over after the formation of the solar system. The large gravity of Jupiter disrupts the formation of a planet, causing an asteroid belt to orbit between Mars and Jupiter.

Consequences of asteroid collision can be:

- craters
- ejection of hot rocks
- widespread fires
- sunlight blocked by dust
- climate change
- species extinction (causing sudden changes of fossil numbers).

A **near-earth object** (NEO) is an asteroid or a comet on a possible collision course with the Earth. An NEO may be seen with telescopes, monitored by satellites and deflected by explosions.

Stars

Stars are giant balls of gas that produce heat and light from nuclear fusion. Here is the life history of a star:

1. Interstellar gas cloud.
2. Gravitational collapse producing a protostar.
3. Thermonuclear fusion.
4. A long period of normal life (**main sequence**).

At the end of its life, the outer layer of a medium-weight star expands to become a **red giant**. It then drifts into space as planetary nebula, leaving a **white dwarf**.

A heavy-weight star also becomes a red giant, then explodes as a **supernova**, then becomes a very dense **neutron star** or a black hole. Our Sun is a medium-weight main sequence star.

A **black hole** has a very large mass and very strong gravity. Nothing can escape from a black hole, not even light.

SUMMARY

- The universe is made up of galaxies, in which there are stars, planets and black holes. There are also smaller bodies called comets, meteorites and asteroids.

- Galileo's observations of Venus proved that Copernicus' heliocentric model of the solar system was incorrect.

- An asteroid or comet on a collision course with Earth is known as a near-earth object (NEO).

- Stars start life as clouds of interstellar dust. They collapse due to gravity, thermonuclear fusion follows and the star enters its main sequence. Depending on the size of the star, it ends its life as either a white dwarf, or a neutron star or black hole.

QUESTIONS

QUICK TEST

1. How often does the Earth rotate?
2. What is the name of our galaxy?
3. What is a red giant?
4. Why can light not escape from a black hole?

EXAM PRACTICE

1. a) Suggest why the geocentric model was accepted for many years. **(2 marks)**

   b) How was Galileo able to gather evidence to disprove the geocentric theory? **(2 marks)**

   c) Suggest what further evidence has allowed us to develop our modern understanding of the solar system. **(3 marks)**

2. Explain why an asteroid belt has formed in our galaxy. **(2 marks)**

3. Describe the life cycle of a star.
   The quality of written communication will be assessed in your answer to this question.
   (6 marks)

Space Exploration

Spacecraft

Extended periods in space can cause deterioration of bones and the heart, and can subject an astronaut to dangerous levels of radiation.

A manned spacecraft must provide:

- enough fuel
- shielding from cosmic rays
- heating and cooling
- artificial gravity
- an air supply
- enough food and water
- exercise machines.

Space travel takes a long time and covers huge distances. **Light years** are used to measure these distances. One light year is the distance light travels in a year.

Unmanned spacecraft can withstand conditions that humans cannot. They have the advantages of cost and safety. However, if something goes wrong, it is difficult to fix. Unmanned spacecraft can collect information on:

- temperature
- magnetic field
- radiation
- gravity
- atmosphere.

Mass, Weight and Force

The **mass** of a body is how much matter it is made of; it does not change. Mass is measured in kilograms (kg). The **weight** of a body is the amount of gravitational **force** acting on it, and can be calculated as follows:

$$\text{Weight (N)} = \text{mass (kg)} \times \text{gravitational field strength (N/kg)}$$

The gravitational field strength (g) is about 9.8 N/kg on Earth.

A spacecraft is powered by ejecting fuel backwards. The **action** of the ejection of fuel backwards causes the **reaction** of the spacecraft forwards. Its motion can be predicted using the equation:

$$\text{Force (N)} = \text{mass (kg)} \times \text{acceleration (m/s}^2)$$

Observations of our Universe

Observations of our universe can be carried out on Earth or in space. Telescopes can detect visible light or other non-visible electromagnetic waves.

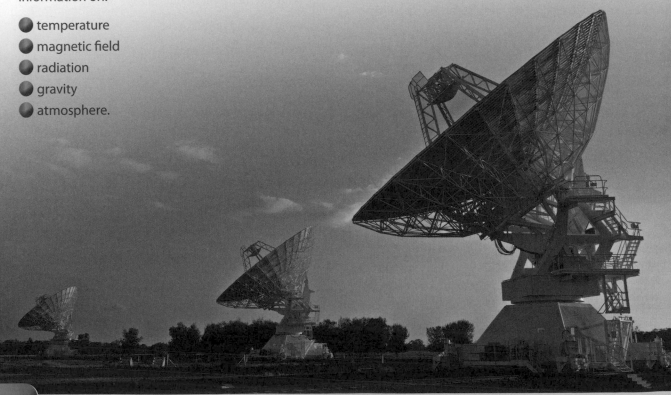

Big Bang Theory

One of the theories of the origin of the universe is that it began with a **Big Bang** from a very small initial point. When galaxies move away from us at high speeds, light waves from them become stretched out, moving their wavelength closer to the red end of the visible spectrum, called '**red-shift**'. The more distant galaxies have a greater red-shift. This means that the galaxies are moving away from each other and the universe is expanding. This supports the Big Bang theory and predicts that the universe began about 15 000 million years ago.

The faint microwave radiation from space, known as **cosmic microwave background radiation**, can be picked up by telescopes and may be left over from the Big Bang.

It is thought that the universe may eventually stop expanding and reach a **steady state**, or that it might eventually collapse and then expand again, **oscillating** continuously.

SUMMARY

- Manned spacecraft require many systems to ensure the astronauts on board remain healthy. Unmanned spacecraft can withstand conditions humans cannot.

- Weight (N) = mass (kg) × $\frac{\text{gravitational field strength (N/kg)}}{}$

- The Big Bang theory is the most widely accepted scientific theory of how the universe began.

- When galaxies move away from us at high speed the light from them is shifted towards the red end of the spectrum. This is known as red-shift.

QUESTIONS

QUICK TEST

1. How can space travel affect the human body?

2. State **three** things a manned spacecraft must provide.

3. What is a light year?

4. Name **three** things that an unmanned spacecraft can collect information about.

EXAM PRACTICE

1. An astronaut has a mass of 80 kg. What would his weight be on:

   a) Earth (g = 9.8 N/kg on Earth)   (1 mark)

   b) The moon (g = 1.6 N/kg on the moon)   (1 mark)

2. The temperature on the surface of Venus is 467 °C and its atmosphere consists of carbon dioxide and nitrogen. Would it be better to use a manned spacecraft or an unmanned probe to explore Venus? Explain your answer.   (3 marks)

3. What evidence is there to support the Big Bang theory?   (4 marks)

Communication

Communication Signals

Mobile phones and satellites use **microwaves** and **radio waves**. Signals can be reflected from the ionosphere or received and re-transmitted by satellites.

Diffraction, refraction and interference around obstacles cause signal loss. This can be reduced by:

- limiting the distance between transmitters
- positioning transmitters as high as possible.

Transmission dishes also experience signal loss due to diffraction.

There have been claims that using mobile phones or living near a phone mast may be dangerous.

Artificial Satellites

Artificial satellites have many different uses, for example:

- telecommunications
- weather prediction
- spying
- satellite navigation systems.

Satellites can be in a polar orbit or a geostationary orbit.

Polar orbit – the satellite passes over both poles whilst the Earth rotates beneath it. The time for one orbit is only a few hours. Weather satellites and spy satellites are in polar orbits.

Geostationary orbit – the satellite stays over the same point on the Earth, so its orbit takes 24 hours. Communication satellites are in geostationary orbits.

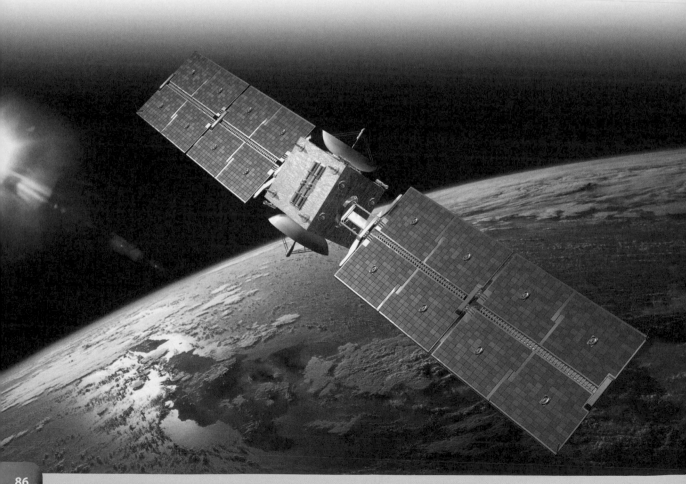

Magnetic Fields

The Earth is surrounded by a **magnetic field**. This is because the Earth's core contains a lot of molten iron. Magnets have a North and a South pole, which can be identified using a plotting compass.

The magnetic field around our planet shields us from much of the ionising radiation from space. An electrical current in a coil also creates a magnetic field.

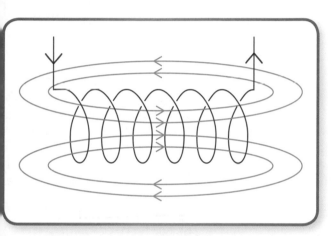

A current flows in the coil (also called a solenoid) producing a magnetic field. The field is the same shape as the field around a bar magnet. As long as the current flows, the coil acts like a bar magnet.

Cosmic Rays and Solar Flares

Cosmic rays causing ionising radiation and **solar flares** from the Sun also interfere with the operation of artificial satellites.

Cosmic rays:

- are fast-moving particles that create gamma rays when they hit the atmosphere
- spiral around the Earth's magnetic field to the poles
- cause the Aurora Borealis and Aurora Australis.

Solar flares:

- are clouds of charged particles from the Sun
- are ejected at high speed
- produce strong disturbances in electromagnetic fields.

QUESTIONS

QUICK TEST

1. What types of waves do mobile phones use?

2. Give two ways that signal loss can be reduced.

3. State two sources of artificial satellite interference.

4. Suggest **two** uses for artificial satellites.

EXAM PRACTICE

1. Why is it important that communication satellites are in geostationary orbits? **(2 marks)**

2. A large mobile phone mast is being built near a school. Some of the parents of children at the school are worried about this, others are not.

   a) Explain why the parents have these two different viewpoints. **(3 marks)**

   b) What evidence could the residents use to help them form an opinion of the safety of the phone mast? **(2 marks)**

3. What benefits do we get from the Earth's magnetic field? **(2 marks)**

Answers

Day 1

pages 4–5
How Science Works

QUICK TEST

1. The variable we choose to change in an experiment
2. The variable that we measure in an experiment
3. A variable that can be put in order
4. A variable that can have any whole-number value
5. Close to the true value

EXAM PRACTICE

1. a) The force applied (1)
   b) The length of the spring (1)
   c) **Accept suitable answers, e.g.** Using the same spring (1).

pages 6–7
Motion

QUICK TEST

1. They need to measure the distance travelled in a certain time.
2. Average velocity $= \dfrac{\text{displacement}}{\text{time}}$
3. 20 m/s (in the direction of travel)
4. Speed has magnitude (size) only; it is a **scalar** quantity. Velocity has magnitude and direction; it is a **vector** quantity.
5. Yes, because the direction changes.

EXAM PRACTICE
1. a) 5.0 m/s^2 (1)
   b) 10 m/s (1)
2. The two trains were travelling in opposite directions (1)
3. The velocity (1) at two different points (1) and the time between them (1)

pages 8–9
Graphs for Motion

QUICK TEST

1. a) i) BC ii) AB iii) CD
   b) 13.3 m/s

EXAM PRACTICE

1. a) 12.5 m/s^2 (1)
   b) Area A–B = 2 × 20 × 0.5 = 20 m; Area B–C = 3 × 20 = 60 m (1); Total distance = 80 m (1)
   c) Max. acceleration C–D (1); $\dfrac{30}{1} = 30$ m/s^2 (1)

pages 10–11
When Forces Combine

QUICK TEST

1. A free body diagram shows the forces that act on a single body.
2. a)
      drag

      weight
   b) 400 N downwards

3. a) He pushes backwards on the boat in order to move forwards.
   b) Action – the man pushes backwards on the boat with a contact force. Reaction – the boat pushes forwards on the man with a contact force.

EXAM PRACTICE

1. a) Friction/drag (1)
   b) 600 N (1)
   c) The forces would be in equilibrium (1); The cyclist would continue at a constant speed if already moving. If the cyclist had stopped he would remain stationary. (1)

pages 12–13
Forces and Motion

QUICK TEST

1. 10 m/s^2
2. Towards the centre
3. Increasing the mass of the body, increasing the speed of the body, or decreasing the radius of the circle

EXAM PRACTICE

1. 90 N (1)
2. $a = \dfrac{60}{30}$ (1); 2 m/s^2 (1)

3. **Key points:**
   - skydiver accelerates
   - due to gravity
   - as speed increases drag increases

- caused by friction
- due to collisions with air particles
- drag = weight (forces balanced)
- terminal velocity
- parachute increases drag
- skydiver decelerates
- decreases drag
- reaches new lower terminal velocity
- lands safely due to low speed

Model answer:
When the skydiver initially jumps from the plane he accelerates due to gravity. As he increases in speed his drag, or friction, from hitting air particles increases. Eventually the force of drag equals the force due to gravity. At this point the skydiver will no longer accelerate but will continue falling at a constant speed. This is terminal velocity. The forces acting on him are balanced. He then deploys his parachute. This increases his drag and so causes him to decelerate. As he decelerates, the force of drag decreases. He will again fall at a constant (though much slower) speed when the force of drag again equals the force due to gravity. This slower speed will allow him to land safely.

pages 14–15
Momentum and Stopping
QUICK TEST
1. 750 kgm/s
2. When a force acts on a body that is moving, or able to move, a change in momentum occurs.
3. Where part of a car is designed to collapse steadily in a collision, spreading stopping over a longer time.
EXAM PRACTICE
1. **a)** 6.0 kgm/s **(1)**   **b)** 3.0 kg **(1)**
   c) 6.0 kgm/s **(1)**
   d) New mass = 3 kg **(1)**,
   New velocity $= \frac{6}{3} = 2.0$ m/s **(1)**

pages 16–17
Day 2
Safe Driving
QUICK TEST
1. The distance travelled between the need for braking occurring and the brakes being applied
2. The distance taken to stop once the brakes have been applied
3. **Any two suitable answers, e.g.** Driver tiredness; Distractions; Lack of concentration
4. If brakes are applied too hard the wheels will lock (stop turning) and the car will begin to skid. ABS braking systems detect this locking and automatically adjust the braking force to prevent skidding.
5. **Any three suitable answers, e.g.** Electric windows; Cruise control; Adjustable seating
EXAM PRACTICE
1. 27 m **(1)**
2. **a)** Braking – Mass of car; Condition of tyres **(1)**. Thinking – Driver alcohol intake; Driver concentration **(1)**.
   b) Concentration is subjective **(1)**; Very difficult to measure – cannot be given a numerical value **(1)**.
3. **Key points:**
   - many factors affect fuel consumption
   - all the factors would have to be controlled in order to make the investigation fair
   - average speed
   - driving style
   - driving style very difficult to quantify
   - the more friction produced the more fuel would be required
   - tyre type and wear would affect friction
   - road conditions would affect friction

Model answer:
There are many different factors that affect a car's fuel consumption. The average speed it was being driven at would have to be calculated. The average style of driving would have to be worked out. This would be very challenging as driving style is a very subjective variable. The tyres on the cars being tested would all need to have the same type and level of tread to ensure the friction they were generating was the same. The road the car was being driven on would have to be the same for each of the test runs. All these variables would have to be controlled before an average fuel consumption could be calculated.

pages 18–19
Energy and Work
QUICK TEST
1. Joules
2. 9 J
3. Increase the object's mass; Increase the object's height; Place it in a stronger gravitational field.
EXAM PRACTICE
1. **a)** Gravitational potential energy **(1)**
   b) 30 000 J **(1)**
   c) 30 000 J **(1)**
   d) $\sqrt{\dfrac{3000}{0.5 \times 100}}$ **(1)**; 24.49 m/s **(1)**

pages 20–21
Work and Power
QUICK TEST
1. Work done is equal to energy transferred; Work is done when a force moves an object
2. **Any two suitable answers, e.g.** Climbing stairs; Pulling a sledge
3. 100 J
4. For an object that is able to recover its original shape, elastic

Answers

potential is the energy stored in the object when work is done to change its shape.

EXAM PRACTICE

1. **a)** 15 000 N **(1)**
   b) 525 000 J **(1)**
   c) 35 000 W **(1)**
   d) 52 500 N weight of load **(1)**;
   $\frac{525\,000}{52\,500} = 10$ m **(1)**

pages 22–23
Static Electricity

QUICK TEST

1. A material that charge (electrons) can pass through
2. A material that charge (electrons) cannot pass through
3. Aircraft fuel causes static charge as the fuel rubs against the pipe. A spark could ignite the fuel vapour. The aircraft and the tanker are earthed to avoid the charge building up.
4. **Any suitable answer, e.g.** Correct earthing; Use of insulating mats
5. **Any suitable answer, e.g.** Synthetic clothing clings; Dirt and dust are attracted to TV screens; Static shocks from cars; Earthed conductors

EXAM PRACTICE

1. **a)** Negatively charged paint **(1)**; Paint droplets repel each other **(1)**; Surface positively charged **(1)**; Paint attracted to surface **(1)**.
   b) The workers could be the route to earth for the static charge on the surface **(1)**.
   c) **Accept one from:** Workers wear rubber-soled shoes; Stand on insulating mats **(1)**.

pages 24–25
Electricity on the Move

QUICK TEST

1. With an ammeter
2. 5.0 C per second
3. **a)** True
   b) False (they flow from negative to positive)

---

   c) False (ions do not move at all)
   d) True

EXAM PRACTICE

1. **a), b)** and **c)** **(3)**

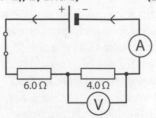

   d) The current will stop flowing **(1)**
2. $\frac{2000}{15}$ **(1)** = 133 Amps **(1)**

pages 26–27
Resistance

QUICK TEST

1. 1.5 Ω
2. It will decrease
3.
4. It would decrease

EXAM PRACTICE

1. **a)** 10 Ω **(1)**
   b) 1.2 A **(1)**
   c) 6.0 V **(1)**
   d) In parallel **(1)**

Day 3

pages 28–29
Electrical Power

QUICK TEST

1. 1.5 W
2. **a)** 240 000 J
   b) 0.067 kWh
3. 4.8 A
4. 96p

EXAM PRACTICE

1. **a)** 144 000 J **(1)**; 0.04 kWh **(1)**
   b) 1 bulb = 9.6p **(1)**
      3 bulbs = 28.8p **(1)**
   c) 0.005 kWh **(1)**
   d) 0.36 kWh **(1)**; 3.6p **(1)**

pages 30–31
Electricity at Home

QUICK TEST

1. The earth wire connects the metal parts of the hairdryer to earth and stops the device

---

becoming dangerous to touch if there is a loose wire. If a large current flows to earth, the fuse melts and breaks the circuit.
2. A residual current circuit breaker. It improves the safety of a device by disconnecting a circuit automatically whenever it detects that the flow of current is too high
3. The resistance of a filament lamp increases with more current – the lamp gets hotter.

EXAM PRACTICE

1. The fuse **(1)**
2. The hair dryer is insulated with a plastic case **(1)** and the wires themselves are also insulated **(1)**
3. It increases **(1)**
4. Current = 3.9 A **(1)**; Fuse would have to be rated higher than this **(1)**
5. **Key points:**
   • current flows in the wire in the bulb
   • electrons collide with ions
   • increases kinetic energy of lattice ions
   • vibrations increase
   • leads to increased collisions
   • this increases the wire's resistance
   • increase in collisions increases temperature
   • as the resistance increases, the current can no longer increase

   Model answer:
   As current flows in the wire in the bulb, electrons collide with ions. This increases the kinetic energy of the lattice ions and causes an increase in vibrations. This leads to further collisions, which leads to an increase in the temperature of the wire and also an increase in its resistance. The increase in resistance prevents the current increasing further.

pages 32–33
Controlling Voltage
QUICK TEST

1.
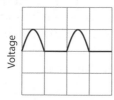

2. Half wave rectification

3. Full wave rectification

4.
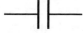

5. To smooth out the current

EXAM PRACTICE

1. **a)** The voltage would increase **(1)**; The capacitor was charging **(1)**.
   b) The voltage would decrease **(1)**; The capacitor was discharging **(1)**.
2. An ordinary resistor would be placed in position R_1 **(1)**; Thermistor in R_2 **(1)**; Cold would increase the resistance of the thermistor **(1)**; This would increase the output voltage **(1)**.

pages 34–35
Electronic Applications
QUICK TEST

1.
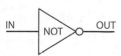

2.

Input	Output
1	0
0	1

3.
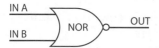

4.

Input A	Input B	Output
0	0	1
0	1	0
1	0	0
1	1	0

5. Any suitable answer, e.g. To switch on the interior light in a car when either the driver's door

or the passenger's door or both doors are open

EXAM PRACTICE

1. High voltage **(1)** and low voltage (0) **(1)**

2.

Input A	Input B	Output
1	0	1
0	1	1
1	1	1
0	0	0	**(4)**

3. It would be the reverse of the above table **(1)**; only 0 on both inputs would give an output of 1 **(1)**.

pages 36–37
Producing Electricity
QUICK TEST

1. It is more efficient – less energy wasted as heat
2. Up to 400 000 V
3. **Any suitable answer, e.g.** They do not spoil the landscape; Protected from the weather.

EXAM PRACTICE

1. **a)** Increasing the strength of the magnet **(1)**. Increasing the number of turns in the coil of wire **(1)**. Increasing the speed of rotation of the coil **(1)**
   b) AC **(1)**
   c) DC is only in one direction **(1)**; AC continuously changes direction **(1)**
   d) Ammeter should be drawn in series with the lamp **(1)**

pages 38–39
Transformers and Motors
QUICK TEST

1. 19 V
2. Increasing the number of turns on the coil; Increasing the current; Using a stronger magnet

EXAM PRACTICE

1. **a)** Primary on left **(1)**; Secondary on right **(1)**
   b) Step-down **(1)**
2. $Vs = \frac{Ns}{Np} \times Vp$ **(1)**; $Vs = 48\,V$ **(1)**

pages 40–41
Electricity in the World
QUICK TEST

1. Increased the processing speed
2. Sending many signals at once
3. It has very little friction
4. The decreasing of resistance to almost zero in certain materials at extremely low temperatures

EXAM PRACTICE

1. An analogue signal is continuously variable **(1)**; A digital signal is either on or off **(1)**
2. A digital signal **(1)**; A digital signal is either on or off so less susceptible to noise **(1)**.
3. Pits store digital information **(1)**; Laser light shone onto surface of CD **(1)**; Light reflected from pits **(1)**; Reflected pulses converted into electrical signal **(1)**.

Day 4

pages 42–43
Harnessing Energy 1
QUICK TEST

1. Chemical energy to heat to kinetic energy (in a turbine that turns a generator) to electrical energy
2. **Any three suitable answers, e.g.** Solar; Wind power; Moving water
3. **Any suitable answer, e.g.** No pollution
4. **Any suitable answer, e.g.** It can disturb habitats
5. Heat to kinetic energy to electrical energy

EXAM PRACTICE

1. fossil, water **(1)**; boiler, turbine **(1)**; turbine, generator **(1)**.
2. Noise pollution **(1)**; Visual pollution **(1)**; Take up large areas of land **(1)**.
3. **Similarities:** Both use water; In both, kinetic energy is converted to electrical energy.

Answers

Differences: Wave power has to be sited by the sea; Hydroelectric power requires a dam to be built; In hydroelectric power, GPE is converted to KE. **(3 marks for any three differences/similarities listed)**

pages 44–45
Harnessing Energy 2
QUICK TEST
1. Requires large areas of land
2. Sulfur dioxide
3. Carbon dioxide
4. CFCs
5. It reflects radiation from the city, which causes warming

EXAM PRACTICE
1. **a)** 25% **(1)**
   b) It is lost as heat **(1)**
2. **a)** 18000 J **(1)**
   b) $\frac{18\,000}{25\,000} \times 100$ **(1)** = 72% **(1)**

pages 46–47
Keeping Warm
QUICK TEST
1. Convection, conduction and radiation
2. Conduction
3. It expands and becomes less dense
4. Matt black
5. **Any three suitable answers, e.g.** Loft insulation; Double glazing; Curtains

EXAM PRACTICE
1. **a)** It is absorbed **(1)**
   b) It is reflected **(1)**
2. **a)** Cavity wall insulation **(1)**
   b) Loft insulation **(1)**; Initial cost is saved in 2 years **(1)**
3. **Key points:**
   • heat loss by conduction
   • reduced by installing double glazing
   • air between glass panes
   • air is a good insulator
   • narrow gap reduces heat loss by convection
   • cavity wall insulation reduces heat loss through walls
   • loft insulation reduces heat lost through roof
   • cavity wall insulation and loft insulation reduce conduction and convection
   • shiny foil reflects heat back into the room from radiators

Model answer:
Heat loss by conduction through windows can be reduced by installing double glazing. The gap between the two panes of glass is filled with air, which is a good insulator. The narrow gap also reduces heat loss by convection. Heat loss through walls can be reduced by using cavity wall insulation. Insulation material is placed inside a gap in the wall, which reduces the heat lost. Fibre glass loft insulation works in a similar way to cavity wall insulation, trapping layers of air between the fibres and reducing heat loss by conduction and convection. Shiny foil can be placed on walls behind radiators to reflect heat energy back into the room.

pages 48–49
Heat
QUICK TEST
1. To absorb more energy
2. A measurement of hotness, measured in degrees Celsius (°C)
3. Heat is a measurement of energy, measured in joules.
4. They have a large surface area compared with their mass so lose heat quickly.
5. Tiles are good thermal conductors and transfer heat away quickly.

EXAM PRACTICE
1. **a)** Can be used in remote locations **(1)**; Low maintenance **(1)**; Produce no waste **(1)**.
   b) Will not work in bad weather **(1)** or at night **(1)**.
2. **a)** Increased distance from light source decreases light intensity **(1)**, so decreases output **(1)**.
   b) Surface area exposed could also affect the output **(1)**.

pages 50–51
Heat Calculations
QUICK TEST
1. The energy needed to increase or decrease the temperature of 1 kg of a material by 1 °C. The unit of specific heat capacity is joules per kg per degree
2. At normal pressure, water freezes and melts at 0 °C
3. The specific latent heat of a substance is the amount of energy required to change the state of 1 kg of that substance at a constant temperature
4. 42 000 J
5. 1925 J

EXAM PRACTICE
1. Mass **(1)**; Material it is made from **(1)**; Temperature change required **(1)**.
2. **a)** Water **(1)**; Has highest specific heat capacity **(1)**.
   b) $2 \times 10 \times 523 = 10\,460$ J **(1)**
3. $330 \times 30 = 9900$ J **(1)**
4. Specific heat capacity $= \frac{30\,000}{(2 \times 6)}$ **(1)**; = 2500 J/kg/°C **(1)**

pages 52–53
Temperature and Pressure
QUICK TEST
1. Temperature is a measure of hotness in degrees Celsius or Kelvin
2. Heat is a measure of energy in joules
3. Absolute zero
4. They stop moving

EXAM PRACTICE
1. 303 Kelvin **(1)**
2. As the temperature decreases, particles have lower kinetic energy so travel slower **(1)**; Impact with cylinder has lower change in momentum **(1)**; Lower frequency of collisions **(1)**.

3. $\frac{230\,000}{323}$ **(1)** $= 712.07 \times 363$ **(1)**
   $= 258\,481$ Pa **(1) (accept answer from 258 481 to 258 483)**

Day 5

pages 54–55
Inside the Atom
QUICK TEST
1. No charge, neutral
2. Huge distances
3. The ability of the radiation to cause other particles to gain or to lose electrons
4. Strong

EXAM PRACTICE
1. **a)** Isotopes **(1)**
   b) 146 **(1)**
   c) $^{238}_{92}\text{U} \rightarrow {}^{234}_{90}\text{Th}$ **(1)** $+ {}^{4}_{2}\alpha$ **(1)**
2. A sheet of aluminium **(1)** a few centimetres thick **(1)** would stop beta and alpha radiation **(1)**.

pages 56–57
Smaller Particles
QUICK TEST
1. The anti-particle to an electron with a positive charge
2. **Any two suitable answers, e.g.** Quarks; Electrons
3. When electrons are 'boiled off' hot metal filaments
4. **Any three suitable answers, e.g.** TV tubes; Oscilloscopes; The production of X-rays
5. By an electric field created by parallel charged metal plates

EXAM PRACTICE
1. **a) b)**

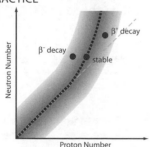

(The β^+ decay can be any point below the curve and β^- decay can be any point above the curve) **(4)**

pages 58–59
Uses of Radiation
QUICK TEST
1. In smoke alarms
2. To find leaks or blockages in underground pipes
3. To limit the exposure and therefore the damage to non-cancerous tissue
4. They are produced in different ways.
5. X-rays are easier to control.

EXAM PRACTICE
1. The time it takes for the number of undecayed nuclei to halve **(1)**
2. **a)** 3 days **(1)**
   b) 50 counts per second **(1)**
3. Energy passed to cathode **(1)**; Cathode loses electrons **(1)**; They are attracted to positive tungsten anode **(1)**; When they hit the tungsten, X-rays are produced **(1)**.

pages 60–61
Dangers of Radiation
QUICK TEST
1. Rocks, cosmic rays and human use (e.g. medical)
2. Yes
3. Thousands of years.
4. It can be encased in glass or concrete and buried.

EXAM PRACTICE
1. They could be concerned about radiation leaks, which could lead to health problems **(1)**, and contaminate the local environment, e.g. affect crops or livestock **(1)**. They could also be concerned about radioactive waste being transported from the plant passing their homes **(1)**.
2. Beta and gamma rays from a source can penetrate the body and cause damage **(1)**; An alpha particle released by an alpha source would be unable to penetrate the body **(1)**.

pages 62–63
Radiation and Science
QUICK TEST
1. If a model is successfully tested, scientists are more likely to accept it.
2. **Any suitable answer, e.g.** Relativity
3. The electron
4. The electrons look a little bit like plums in a pudding.
5. Electrons can behave like clouds of charge, or even waves.

EXAM PRACTICE
1. Other scientists must be able to use the same method **(1)**; To produce the same results (show that the experiment is repeatable) **(1)**; So that the theory can be accepted as fact **(1)**.
2. **a)** Must be lots of empty space as most alpha particles do not come into contact with anything **(1)** and pass straight through **(1)**.
   b) Very few particles are deflected a lot by the positive charge of the nucleus **(1)** which repels the positively charged alpha particles **(1)**.

pages 64–65
Nuclear Power
QUICK TEST
1. Two lighter nuclei and two or three neutrons
2. The two lighter nuclei
3. The joining of two atomic nuclei to form a larger (heavier) one

EXAM PRACTICE
1. When a neutron hits the uranium 235 atom, the atom splits and releases neutrons **(1)**. These neutrons can hit other uranium 235 atoms **(1)**, causing these atoms to also split and further neutrons to be released, and so on **(1)**.

Answers

2. Requires very high temperatures and pressures **(1)**; More energy is required than is produced **(1)**.

3. **Key points:**
   - uranium 235 undergoes nuclear fission
   - when a neutron hits the uranium 235 atom, the atom splits and releases neutrons
   - these neutrons can hit other uranium 235 atoms
   - a chain reaction occurs
   - this produces a large amount of heat
   - heat is used to boil water in a boiler
   - high pressure steam is produced
   - steam then flows over a turbine
   - turbine blades turn
   - turbine is connected to a generator
   - generator produces an electric current

Model answer:
Uranium 235, or some other nuclear fuel, undergoes nuclear fission. This produces a large amount of heat, which is used to boil water in a boiler. This produces high pressure steam. The steam then flows over a turbine, turning its blades. The turbine is connected to a generator. The turning of the turbine blades causes the generator to produce electricity.

Day 6

pages 66–67
Waves
QUICK TEST

1. Wavelength is the distance between any point on a wave and the same point on the next wave.
2. Amplitude is the maximum displacement of the waves from rest position.
3. The total time taken for a single wave to pass a point
4. Longitudinal

---

5. Transverse
EXAM PRACTICE
1. 4 Hz **(1)**
2. 1.32 m **(1)**
3. **Key points:**
   - P-waves are longitudinal waves, which travel through solids and liquids
   - P-waves are detected on the opposite sides of the Earth to a quake
   - S-waves are transverse waves that travel through solid rock only
   - S-waves are not detected on the opposite side of the Earth to a quake
   - this suggests that at least part of the Earth's core is liquid
   - P- and S-waves are detected at points on the Earth's surface not directly opposite the epicentre
   - this is due to refraction
   - suggests the mantle is solid rock
   - suggests the mantle has different densities, which causes the refraction

Model answer:
P-waves are longitudinal waves, which can travel through solids and liquids. S-waves are transverse waves, which travel through solid rock only. P-waves are detected on the opposite side of the Earth to the epicentre of a quake, whereas S-waves are not. This suggests that the Earth has a liquid core. Both P-waves and S-waves are detected at points on the Earth's surface, which are not directly opposite the epicentre. This suggests that around the core there is the mantle, consisting of solid rock of differing densities, which refracts the waves as they travel through it.

---

pages 68–69
Reflection
QUICK TEST

1. Angle of incidence = Angle of reflection
2. Virtual, upright, same size as the object
3. A constructed line perpendicular to any reflecting surface at the point where the incident ray hits the surface

EXAM PRACTICE
1. A real image can be focused on a screen **(1)**; A virtual image cannot **(1)** – you have to look into the mirror to see it **(1)**
2. **a)** Object must be between C and F **(1)**
   b) Object must be closer than F **(1)**
   c) Object must be beyond C **(1)**

pages 70–71
Wave Behaviour 1
QUICK TEST

1. Lines drawn one wavelength apart, perpendicular to the direction of the waves
2. Areas where the waves add together (reinforcement)
3. An even number of half wavelengths (i.e. a whole number of waves)
4. No
5. Sunglasses / camera lens

EXAM PRACTICE
1. The spreading out of waves when they pass through a gap **(1)**
2. It stays the same **(1)**
3. **a)**

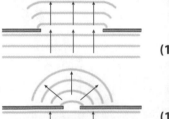

(1)

(1)

   b) The size of the gap must be similar to the wavelength **(1)** for diffraction to be significant **(1)**.

pages 72–73
Wave Behaviour 2
QUICK TEST
1. When a wave changes direction as it travels from one medium to another
2. When it leaves water and enters air
3. Because of apparent depth due to refraction
4. When a narrow beam of white light passes through a prism it separates into a spectrum of colour due to refraction
5. Sending many signals along an optical fibre at once

EXAM PRACTICE
1. a) Total internal reflection **(1)**
   b)
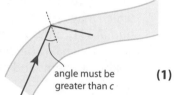
angle must be greater than *c* **(1)**

   c)
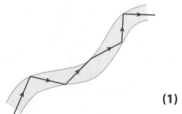
(1)

2. a) Different wavelengths of light are slowed down by different amounts as they enter the prism **(1)**; The higher the refractive index **(1)**, the greater the refraction **(1)**.
   b) Blue **(1)**; It has the higher refractive index **(1)**.

pages 74–75
Lenses
QUICK TEST
1. Real, inverted, the same size as the object
2. **Any two from:** Upright; Virtual; Smaller than the object

EXAM PRACTICE
1. **Any three from:** Cameras; Magnifying glasses; Projectors; Glasses **(3)**.

2. 8 × magnification **(1)**
3. $\frac{26}{78}$ **(1)** = 0.33 m **(1)**

pages 76–77
The Eye
QUICK TEST
1.
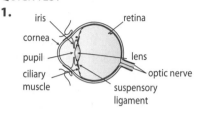

2. Short-sightedness is caused by the eyeball being too long; Long-sightedness is caused by the eyeball being too short; Both can also be caused by the lens being unable to focus.
3. Both use a lens to focus light on a light-sensitive area

EXAM PRACTICE
1. a) Ciliary muscles contract **(1)**; Lens becomes fatter **(1)**; Light is refracted more and focused on retina **(1)**
   b) Ciliary muscles relax **(1)**; Lens becomes thinner **(1)**; Light is refracted less and focused on retina **(1)**
2. a) Light from near object is not being focused on retina **(1)**; Light is not being refracted enough **(1)**.
   b) Glasses or contact lenses could be worn **(1)**; Laser surgery could be carried out **(1)**; All of these methods would increase refraction of light **(1)** leading to the light being focused on the retina **(1)**

Day 7
pages 78–79
The Electromagnetic Spectrum
QUICK TEST
1. The type of radiation and the size of the dose
2. It may kill the cells

3. **Any suitable answer, e.g.** Ultraviolet light to detect forged bank notes
4. **Any suitable answer, e.g.** Optical waves for iris recognition
5. **Any suitable answer, e.g.** Infrared to monitor temperature

EXAM PRACTICE
1. **Any suitable answer, e.g.** Ultraviolet **(1)**, X-rays **(1)** and gamma rays **(1)**.
2. 1400 x 4 = 5600 **(1)**; $\frac{5600}{2}$ = 2800 m **(1)**
3. Most of the microwaves are absorbed by water and fat particles in the outer layer of the food **(1)**; This increases their kinetic energy **(1)**; This kinetic energy is transferred to the centre of the food by conduction or convection **(1)**.

pages 80–81
Sound
QUICK TEST
1. Ultrasound
2. Larger amplitude makes a louder sound
3. Higher frequency makes a higher pitch/note

EXAM PRACTICE
1. a) In a sound wave the particles vibrate backwards and forwards **(1)**; Parallel to the direction of the wave **(1)**.
   b) A microphone detects the sound waves **(1)**; An oscilloscope translates the vibrations into an image of a transverse wave **(1)**.
2. It can produce images of soft tissues **(1)**; It does not damage living cells **(1)**.
3. Pitch and loudness are independent **(1)**; It is possible to have a loud sound that is high or low pitched **(1)** or a quiet sound that is high or low pitched **(1)**.

Answers

pages 82–83
Beyond our Planet
QUICK TEST
1. Every 24 hours
2. The Milky Way
3. A star that has expanded outer layers near the end of its life
4. Because of the very strong gravity

EXAM PRACTICE
1. a) **Any two from:** The church was very influential and believed the Earth was the centre of the universe; The Sun seemed to move across the sky; Technology did not exist to gather more evidence (**2**).
   b) He developed the first telescope (**1**), which allowed him to view Venus closely enough to observe features of its orbit (**1**).
   c) Newton's theory of gravity (**1**); More powerful telescopes (**1**); Space probes (**1**).
2. The large gravity of Jupiter (**1**) disrupts the normal formation of a planet between Jupiter and Mars (**1**).
3. **Key points:**
   • an interstellar cloud of gas
   • collapses
   • due to gravity
   • forms a protostar
   • thermonuclear fusion occurs
   • star is now in its main sequence
   • this can last for billions of years
   • at the end of its life, star forms a red giant
   • medium-weight star then forms a white dwarf
   • heavy-weight star explodes in a supernova
   • releases large amounts of dust and gas
   • forms a neutron star
   • or a black hole

Model answer:
An interstellar cloud of gas collapses under its own gravity and forms a protostar. Thermonuclear fusion occurs in the protostar and the star enters its main sequence, which can last for billions of years. At the end of its life, a star expands to become a red giant. A medium-weight star will then contract and cool to form a white dwarf. A heavy-weight star will explode in a supernova, releasing dust and gas. It will then either form a neutron star or a black hole.

pages 84–85
Space Exploration
QUICK TEST
1. It can cause deterioration of bones and of the heart
2. **Any three suitable answers, e.g.** Artificial gravity; Air supply; Enough food and water
3. The distance light travels in a year
4. **Any three suitable answers, e.g.** Temperature; Magnetic field; Atmosphere

EXAM PRACTICE
1. a) 784 N (**1**)
   b) 128 N (**1**)
2. An unmanned probe (**1**); Temperature and atmospheric conditions (**1**) would make it very hostile and dangerous for humans (**1**).
3. Cosmic microwave background radiation (**1**); Galaxies are moving away from us (**1**); Evidence for this is red-shift (**1**); Light from them is shifted to the red end of the spectrum (**1**).

pages 86–87
Communication
QUICK TEST
1. Microwaves and radio waves
2. Limiting the distance between transmitters; Positioning transmitters as high as possible
3. Cosmic rays causing ionising radiation and solar flares from the Sun
4. **Any two suitable answers, e.g.** Spying; Satellite navigation systems

EXAM PRACTICE
1. So that they can receive and send signals (**1**) from the area they are covering (**1**).
2. a) Mobile phone masts use microwave radiation (**1**); which may be harmful to humans (**1**); although there is no proven link between health problems and mobile phone masts (**1**).
   b) Check the results of published scientific surveys (**1**) into the effects of phone masts on children's health (**1**).
3. Allows us to navigate using a compass (**1**); Protects us from cosmic rays (**1**).